A MATTER OF SIZE

TRIENNIAL REVIEW OF THE NATIONAL NANOTECHNOLOGY INITIATIVE

Committee to Review the National Nanotechnology Initiative

National Materials Advisory Board

Division on Engineering and Physical Sciences

NATIONAL RESEARCH COUNCIL
OF THE NATIONAL ACADEMIES

THE NATIONAL ACADEMIES PRESS
Washington, D.C.
www.nap.edu

THE NATIONAL ACADEMIES PRESS • 500 Fifth Street, N.W. • Washington, DC 20001

NOTICE: The project that is the subject of this report was approved by the Governing Board of the National Research Council, whose members are drawn from the councils of the National Academy of Sciences, the National Academy of Engineering, and the Institute of Medicine. The members of the committee responsible for the report were chosen for their special competences and with regard for appropriate balance.

This report is based on work supported by the National Science Foundation under Grant No. CTS-0436444. Any opinions, findings, and conclusions or recommendations expressed in this material are those of the author(s) and do not necessarily reflect the views of the National Science Foundation.

International Standard Book Number-10: 0-309-10223-5
International Standard Book Number-13: 978-0-309-10223-0

Cover: Clockwise from top right:

- "Flower Bouquet," a three-dimensional nanostructure grown by controlled nucleation of silicon carbide nanowires on gallium catalyst particles. © Ghim Wei Ho and Mark Welland, University of Cambridge. Reprinted with permission.
- Scanning electron microscopy image of chemical vapor deposition synthesis of carbon nanotubes. Courtesy of NASA.
- Array of vertically aligned carbon nanotubes grown using plasma-enhanced chemical vapor deposition, which is then intercalated with copper to create a composite exhibiting good thermal properties applicable for chip cooling. Courtesy of NASA.
- Scanning electron microscopy image of hexagonal zinc oxide nanocrystallites. Courtesy of the National Science Foundation and Yicheng Lu, Sriram Muthukumar, and Nuri Emanetoglu, Rutgers University.
- Scanning electron microscopy image of zinc oxide nanowires grown on silicon in which the average width of the rods is 40 to 50 nanometers. Courtesy of the National Science Foundation and Yicheng Lu, Sriram Muthukumar, and Nuri Emanetoglu, Rutgers University.
- "Nano Rings" grown by varying the conditions of chemical vapor deposition synthesis of silicon composite nanostructures. © Ghim Wei Ho and Mark Welland, University of Cambridge. Reprinted with permission.
- "Transport XI," part of a series on electron transport in semiconductors, shows electrons that are launched over a very small range of initial angles, represented by the narrow "stems." Small initial differences in angle grow quickly, as evidenced by the fanning out and branching of electron paths. © Eric J. Heller, Harvard University. Reprinted with permission.
- Scanning electron microscopy image of an array of carbon nanotubes grown by chemical vapor deposition. Courtesy of NASA.

Copies of this report are available from the National Academies Press, 500 Fifth Street, N.W., Lockbox 285, Washington, DC 20055; (800) 624-6242 or (202) 334-3313 (in the Washington metropolitan area); Internet, http://www.nap.edu.

Additional copies of this report are available from:

National Materials Advisory Board
500 Fifth Street, N.W.
Washington, DC 20001
nmab@nas.edu
http://www.nas.edu/nmab

THE NATIONAL ACADEMIES
Advisers to the Nation on Science, Engineering, and Medicine

The **National Academy of Sciences** is a private, nonprofit, self-perpetuating society of distinguished scholars engaged in scientific and engineering research, dedicated to the furtherance of science and technology and to their use for the general welfare. Upon the authority of the charter granted to it by the Congress in 1863, the Academy has a mandate that requires it to advise the federal government on scientific and technical matters. Dr. Ralph J. Cicerone is president of the National Academy of Sciences.

The **National Academy of Engineering** was established in 1964, under the charter of the National Academy of Sciences, as a parallel organization of outstanding engineers. It is autonomous in its administration and in the selection of its members, sharing with the National Academy of Sciences the responsibility for advising the federal government. The National Academy of Engineering also sponsors engineering programs aimed at meeting national needs, encourages education and research, and recognizes the superior achievements of engineers. Dr. Wm. A. Wulf is president of the National Academy of Engineering.

The **Institute of Medicine** was established in 1970 by the National Academy of Sciences to secure the services of eminent members of appropriate professions in the examination of policy matters pertaining to the health of the public. The Institute acts under the responsibility given to the National Academy of Sciences by its congressional charter to be an adviser to the federal government and, upon its own initiative, to identify issues of medical care, research, and education. Dr. Harvey V. Fineberg is president of the Institute of Medicine.

The **National Research Council** was organized by the National Academy of Sciences in 1916 to associate the broad community of science and technology with the Academy's purposes of furthering knowledge and advising the federal government. Functioning in accordance with general policies determined by the Academy, the Council has become the principal operating agency of both the National Academy of Sciences and the National Academy of Engineering in providing services to the government, the public, and the scientific and engineering communities. The Council is administered jointly by both Academies and the Institute of Medicine. Dr. Ralph J. Cicerone and Dr. Wm. A. Wulf are chair and vice chair, respectively, of the National Research Council.

www.national-academies.org

COMMITTEE TO REVIEW THE
NATIONAL NANOTECHNOLOGY INITIATIVE

JAMES C. WILLIAMS, Ohio State University, *Chair*
CHERRY A. MURRAY, Lawrence Livermore National Laboratory, *Vice Chair*
A. MICHAEL ANDREWS II, L3 Communications Corporation
MARK J. CARDILLO, The Camille and Henry Dreyfus Foundation
CRYSTAL CUNANAN, ReVision Optics, Inc.
PETER H. DIAMANDIS, X PRIZE Foundation
PAUL A. FLEURY, Yale University
PAUL B. GERMERAAD, Intellectual Assets, Inc.
ALAN H. GOLDSTEIN, Alfred University
MARY L. GOOD, University of Arkansas at Little Rock
THOMAS S. HARTWICK, TRW, Inc. (retired)
MAYNARD A. HOLLIDAY, Evolution Robotics, Inc.
RICHARD L. IRVING, Lakewood Village Community Church, Long Beach, California
DONALD H. LEVY, James Franck Institute, University of Chicago
BETTIE SUE MASTERS, University of Texas Health Science Center at San Antonio
SONIA E. MILLER, Converging Technologies Bar Association
EDWARD K. MORAN, Deloitte & Touche USA LLP
DAVID C. MOWERY, Walter A. Haas School of Business, University of California, Berkeley
KATHLEEN M. REST, Union of Concerned Scientists
THOMAS A. SAPONAS, Agilent Technologies (retired)
R. PAUL SCHAUDIES, Science Applications International Corporation
TSUNG-TSAN SU, NanoTechnology Research Center, Industrial Technology Research Institute, Taiwan
THOMAS N. THEIS, IBM Thomas J. Watson Research Center

Staff

GARY FISCHMAN, National Materials Advisory Board (NMAB), Director
DENNIS CHAMOT, Division on Engineering and Physical Sciences, Acting NMAB Director
TONI MARECHAUX, Board on Manufacturing and Engineering Design, Past Director
MICHAEL H. MOLONEY, Senior Program Officer

TAMAE MAEDA WONG, Senior Program Officer
EUGENE J. CHOI, Program Officer
TERI THOROWGOOD, Administrative Coordinator
COLLEEN BRENNAN, Program Associate
LAURA TOTH, Senior Program Assistant

NATIONAL MATERIALS ADVISORY BOARD

Preface

The National Research Council (NRC) was asked by the U.S. Congress to conduct the first triennial evaluation of the National Nanotechnology Initiative (NNI);[1] assess the need for standards, guidelines, or strategies for ensuring the responsible development of nanotechnology; and consider the technical feasibility of molecular self-assembly for the manufacture of materials and devices at the molecular scale. The full statement of task is given in Appendix A.

APPROACH TO AND SCOPE OF THIS STUDY

To conduct this study, the NRC appointed the Committee to Review the National Nanotechnology Initiative, whose members' expertise ranged from nanoscale science and engineering to industrial research and development (R&D) and encompassed interdisciplinary research, business management, biomedicine and human health, public and environmental safety, national defense, international benchmarking, transfer of technology for commercialization, intellectual property issues, and the societal and ethical implications of nanotechnology; see Appendix B.

To gather information on and gain insight into the multiagency collaborations and extensive R&D programs associated with the NNI, the committee held a series of public workshops participated in by members of the broader NNI-related com-

---

[1]A review of the National Nanotechnology Initiative by the NRC in 2002 was published in *Small Wonders, Endless Frontiers: A Review of the National Nanotechnology Initiative* (National Academy Press, Washington, D.C., 2002).

munity, including representatives of the federal agencies participating in the NNI. The meeting and workshop agendas along with lists of participants are provided in Appendix C. Summaries of the presentations made at the workshop on responsible development are presented in Appendix D. Appendix E defines the acronyms used in the report. In addition to its four workshops the committee held a series of closed private sessions and telephone conferences to discuss its findings and to develop its conclusions and recommendations.

Given the length and breadth of its charge (see Appendix A), the committee sought an approach that would give an accurate picture of the NNI and its accomplishments today and also allow identification of opportunities for improvement in the future (Chapter 1), as well as enable assessment of the relative position of U.S. nanotechnology R&D compared to that of other nations (Chapter 2) and a discussion of the impact of nanotechnology on the U.S. economy (Chapter 3). The complexity and detail of the set of programmatic tasks and the quite different requirements posed by the two additional tasks, on the responsible development of nanotechnology (Chapter 4) and molecular self-assembly (Chapter 5), added considerable complexity to the task. To provide a useful analysis, the committee focused only on topics accessible to examination and for which at least some reliable data were available. It notes that—considered in light of the major benefits anticipated—the NNI represents a comparatively young undertaking whose results will take time to develop, and also to measure quantitatively. Although the committee's treatment of the many topics in its charge is uneven, it dealt with each to the extent possible, except as noted below.

In its discussion of both the relative position of the United States worldwide in nanoscale R&D and the economic impact of nanotechnology, the committee chose to consider not only NNI-related R&D, but also research supported by private and public funds, as well as research supported by federal funds not associated with the NNI, given that nanotechnology R&D is being conducted at industrial R&D laboratories and that sources of support for nanotechnology R&D also include private foundations and venture capital funds—and that isolating the contributions of each was beyond the committee's ability to accomplish for this study.

With respect to responsible development of nanotechnology, the committee focused on tangible concerns related to environmental, health, and safety issues and also touched on the importance of broadly targeted efforts in communication on and education about societal concerns. As a result of its reflections on and discussion of what is regarded as the more futuristic aspects of nanotechnology—such as the use of nanotechnology in developing artificial intelligence, and similar topics popularized in science fiction—the committee decided that an assessment of such topics in the context of a need for standards and guidelines would be premature and speculative at best. Therefore, the committee chose to address potential real risks rather than perceived risks pertaining to nanotechnology. The committee points out that several interesting observations on societal implications are presented in the individually authored signed summaries of presentations made at its Workshop on Responsible Development of Nanotechnology (see Appendix D). The committee is convinced that delineating and addressing the kinds of issues raised by such observations is critical to realizing the full potential of nanotechnology.

This study does not include a comprehensive technical assessment of the NNI to date, beyond the benchmarking and examination of economic impact reported in Chapters 2 and 3. The committee was hampered in its efforts by a number of things: the interdisciplinary nature of nanotechnology R&D, which includes a mix of the physical sciences, engineering, technology, and biomedical sciences; the impossibility of isolating and measuring the contributions of individual nanoscale R&D programs; the long timescales needed to translate to practical benefits the results of nanoscale R&D that is still in its infancy; and the enormous technical breadth of the approximately $1.1 billion in R&D carried out annually. However, the committee did receive anecdotal evidence of significant achievements across many fields, including information presented at its workshop on scientific achievements, and makes reference to some of those at points in the report. The committee is convinced that the R&D infrastructure now being developed under the NNI will help make possible technical achievements whose impact will become apparent and amenable to study, over time.

In addition, the committee did not attempt to assess the funding levels at each NNI-participating agency in terms of their adequacy for meeting stated program goals. Such an evaluation would have required a program by program analysis of each agency—an effort beyond the committee's resources and one also precluded by the lack of consistent reporting and tracking of funds requested, authorized, and expended within and across agencies. The committee reiterates, moreover, that it is too early to fully assess, at this early stage in nanoscale R&D, technical accomplishments and goals achieved as a result of investments made under the NNI.

ACKNOWLEDGMENTS

To better calibrate the data presented in the workshops, individual committee members contacted corporate leaders in various nanotechnology sectors and operations, from start-up companies to multinational corporations, to seek an industry perspective on commercial nanotechnologies, nanotechnology R&D, and NNI programs. In this regard the committee is grateful to the following participants in that process: Larry Bock, Nanosys; Uma Chowdhry and Krishna Doraiswamy, DuPont; Daniel Gamota, Motorola; Paolo Gargini, Intel Corporation;

Michael Helmus and Magnus Gittins, Advance Nanotech; Michael Idelchik, GE Global Research; Amit Kumar, CombiMatrix Corp.; David Macdonald, Nanomix; Hash Pakbaz, Cambrios Technologies Corp.; and Sharon Smith, Lockheed Martin Corporation.

In addition, the committee acknowledges with thanks the active participation of NNI agency representatives, nanoscience researchers, industrial technologists, and health professionals in its information-gathering efforts. The committee thanks in particular NSET Subcommittee representatives Celia Merzbacher, James Murday, Mihail Roco, and Clayton Teague and their staffs for their willingness to provide every possible assistance in the course of this study. The input from and willingness of the broad nanotechnology community to contribute to enhancing the committee's understanding of the diverse issues are greatly appreciated. The committee also thanks those who submitted written material and provided comments at the committee's workshops and open meetings. Thanks are also due to Mark Welland for his input and counsel provided in his role as consultant to the committee.

The committee thanks NRC staff members Dennis Chamot, Gary Fischman, Toni Marechaux, Tamae Maeda Wong, Michael Moloney, Eugene J. Choi, Colleen Brennan, Teri Thorowgood, Laura Toth, and Heather Lozowski for their advice and efforts during this study. It also notes the contributions from the following young scientists who were assigned to assist the committee through the National Academies' Christine Mirzayan Science and Technology Policy Fellowship Program: Rachel Fezzie, Benjamin Gross, Nagesh Rao, and Shara Williams. The committee was also fortunate to have the help of Scott Martindale, a science and journalism student at the University of Southern California. Finally, the committee thanks Terry Lowe, who acted as a liaison from the National Materials Advisory Board, of which he is a member, for his critical guidance to the committee in the execution of its charge.

Jim Williams, *Chair*
Cherry Murray, *Vice Chair*
Committee to Review the National Nanotechnology Initiative

Acknowledgment of Reviewers

This report has been reviewed in draft form by individuals chosen for their diverse perspectives and technical expertise, in accordance with procedures approved by the National Research Council's (NRC's) Report Review Committee. The purpose of this independent review is to provide candid and critical comments that will assist the institution in making its published report as sound as possible and to ensure that the report meets institutional standards for objectivity, evidence, and responsiveness to the study charge. The review comments and draft manuscript remain confidential to protect the integrity of the deliberative process. We wish to thank the following individuals for their review of this report:

Ashish Arora, Carnegie Mellon University,
William F. Brinkman, Princeton University,
Douglas Daugherty, ENVIRON,
Judith Ann Graham, American Chemistry Council,
Philippe Guyot-Sionnest, University of Chicago,
Evelyn L. Hu, University of California, Santa Barbara,
William J. Madia, Battelle Memorial Institute,
Stephen B. Maebius, Foley & Lardner LLP,
Thomas J. Meyer, University of North Carolina, Chapel Hill,
David Scheinberg, Sloan-Kettering Institute,
Paul S. Weiss, Pennsylvania State University, and
George Whitesides, Harvard University.

Although the reviewers listed above have provided many constructive comments and suggestions, they were not asked to endorse the conclusions or recommendations, nor did they see the final draft of the report before its release. The review of this report was overseen by Pierre C. Hohenberg, New York University, and Julia R. Weertman, Northwestern University. Appointed by the NRC, they were responsible for making certain that an independent examination of this report was carried out in accordance with institutional procedures and that all review comments were carefully considered. Responsibility for the final content of this report rests entirely with the authoring committee and the institution.

Contents

Summary

Nanoscale science, engineering, and technology can be characterized as sets of fundamental knowledge and enabling technologies derived from efforts to understand and control the properties and function of matter at the nanoscale dimension—that is, at a scale on the order of one-billionth of a meter, or approximately 1/100,000th of the width of a strand of human hair. The National Nanotechnology Initiative (NNI), a federal interagency activity established in 2000, aims to expedite the discovery, development, and deployment of nanotechnology in order to achieve responsible and sustainable economic benefits, enhance the quality of life, and promote national security. Requested by Congress (see Appendix A), this report of the National Research Council's Committee to Review the National Nanotechnology Initiative is an evaluation of the NNI that also considers the current economic impact of nanotechnology and benchmarks the international standing of U.S. nanoscale research and development (R&D). In addition, the report addresses the responsible development of nanotechnology and comments on the feasibility of molecular self-assembly for manufacturing.

THE NNI TODAY

It is important to note that the NNI is not a government research program per se, since it does not distribute research support to individual scientists or R&D centers and consortia. Rather, the NNI is a mechanism, mandated at the highest levels of government, for the coordination of federal research interests in nanotechnology. Established in 2000, the NNI is relatively young, especially when viewed from the perspective of the typical timescales needed to reap the benefits of research on an emerging technology. The 20- to 40-year period for the development of computing and communications technologies made possible by basic research funded earlier in the 20th century offers an apt comparison. A basic tenet of the committee's analysis is that the NNI clearly represents a long-term undertaking whose goals and benefits will take time to realize. Moreover, nanotechnology is an enabling technology whose impact may be difficult to determine fully and rigorously even as the technology matures and appears in widely available products. In this report, the committee (1) discusses accomplishments of the NNI to date that augur well for ongoing progress in nanotechnology R&D to benefit the nation and (2) offers recommendations aimed at ensuring an enhanced U.S. capacity to realize and measure discernible benefits, responsibly developed, from nanoscale R&D into the future.

NNI Structure and Goals

The NNI has several management layers that are described in detail in Chapter 1. In summary, the National Science and Technology Council, a cabinet-level committee with a membership drawn from federal agencies across the government, through its Committee on Technology formed the Nanoscale Science, Engineering, and Technology (NSET) Subcommittee to focus on NNI activities. The NSET Subcommittee currently involves more than 20 federal agencies. In FY 2005, 11 agencies reported investments in nanotechnology under the NNI umbrella that totaled about $1.1 billion.[1] The National Nanotechnology Coordination Office (NNCO), established in 2001, provides technical guidance and administrative support to the NSET Subcommittee, facilitates multiagency planning, conducts activities and workshops, and prepares information and reports. In addition, in 2004 the President's Council of Advisors on Science and Technology (PCAST) was designated by President George W. Bush as the National Nanotechnology Advisory Panel (NNAP).[2] Chapter 1 discusses the role of the NNAP in more detail.

The NNI has four goals:[3]

- Goal 1: Maintain a world-class research and development program aimed at realizing the full potential of nanotechnology.
- Goal 2: Facilitate transfer of new technologies into products for economic growth, jobs, and other public benefit.
- Goal 3: Develop educational resources, a skilled workforce, and the supporting infrastructure and tools to advance nanotechnology.
- Goal 4: Support responsible development of nanotechnology.

In pursuit of these goals, the NNI has defined seven program component areas (PCAs) that provide a framework by which the participating agencies can better direct, coordinate, and report on their activities.[4] As well as supplying coordinating mechanisms, the NNI also provides a forum for research agencies to discuss cross-cutting science and policy issues related to the development of nanotechnology.

NNI Accomplishments and Impacts

Notwithstanding the extensive and detailed charge for this study (see Appendix A); the many layers to and multiple participants in the operation of the NNI (see Figure 1-1 in Chapter 1); the fact that data on NNI-related activities, if reported at all, are not reported in a self-consistent manner across the federal agencies; and the breadth and diversity of the science that falls under the umbrella of the NNI, the committee carried out a review of the NNI that focused on assessing the NNI's progress toward meeting its stated goals and outlining the NNI's achievements to date. The data gathered in the benchmarking and economic impact parts of the study as detailed in Chapter 2 and Chapter 3, respectively, and presentations made at the committee's workshop on scientific accomplishments gave valuable insight into the positive effects of the NNI. The committee's analysis and the supporting information gathered during this study are summarized here and provided in more detail in the main body of the report.

NNI Coordination and Its Results

Established to enhance dialog and coordination across nanoscale R&D programs at federal agencies, the NNI has facilitated the following developments,[5] among others:

- Establishment by the NSET Subcommittee of four interagency working groups—Nanotechnology Environmental and Health Implications (NEHI); Industry Liaison; Manufacturing; and Nanotechnology Public Engagement—that have promoted cross-agency collaboration such as joint work in manufacturing technologies by the Department of Defense (DOD) and the National Science Foundation (NSF), and in explosive vapor detection by the Department of Energy (DOE) and DOD, to name a few, and have facilitated communication among agency officials who might otherwise not have had the opportunity to meet and discover shared interests;
- Development of the NSF National Nanotechnology Infrastructure Network, an integrated partnership of user facilities at 13 campuses across the United States whose mission is to enable rapid advances in nanotechnology

by providing efficient access to facilities for fabrication, synthesis, and characterization;[6]

- Development of the DOE's network of five new nanoscale science and engineering centers designed to support synthesis, processing, fabrication, and analysis at the nanoscale;[7]
- An abundance of interdisciplinary activity in NNI-related programs, broadening the direction of some research at federal agencies, such as research in the Program of Excellence in Nanotechnology at the National Heart, Lung, and Blood Institute;
- Establishment of several NNI-industry consultative boards to facilitate networking and partnerships among R&D organizations, industry sectors, and government agencies;[8]
- Policy impacts at the state level as a result of increased coordination at the federal level, such as establishment in 2000 of the California NanoSystems Institute, in which the state of California invested $100 million and federal and industry funds totaled $250 million, to provide a multidisciplinary environment in materials science, molecular electronics, quantum computing, optical networking, and molecular medicine designed to stimulate crosscutting nanoscale R&D;
- Programmatic and budget redirection within agencies attributable to NNI coordination outcomes, such as the FY 2005 refocusing of the Environmental Protection Agency's nanotechnology resources on studies of the toxicity of nanomaterials; and
- Establishment by the NNI-participating agencies of joint programs and exploration of new paradigms for federal investments, despite recent funding constraints and little new R&D funding over the last few years. In some NNI agencies the process of strategic planning and identifying the seven PCAs has been important for engaging the interest of and securing support from various intra-agency components for nanoscale R&D programs.

In summary, considerable evidence indicates that the NNI is successfully coordinating nanoscale R&D efforts and interests across the federal government; catalyzing cooperative research and technology development across a spectrum of disciplines from engineering and the physical sciences to biosciences and biomedicine; and opening a host of new opportunities for scientific discoveries at the nanoscale with, for example, a suite of nanoscale national facilities, laboratories, and research support programs (see Box 1-3 in Chapter 1 for some examples of NNI-related centers). In addition, the NNI-participating agencies have made significant progress toward establishing a national R&D infrastructure to support innovation at the nanoscale, as detailed in Chapter 1. Much of this operational success has been enabled by the effective communication and coordination fostered by the NSET Subcommittee and the NNCO. The committee thus concluded that increased interagency coordination—which has enhanced the development of interdisciplinary research, led to improvements in the R&D infrastructure, and stimulated new areas in research—is an important impact of the NNI.

Benchmarking of U.S. International Standing and Economic Impact of Nanotechnology R&D

As discussed in more detail in Chapter 2, benchmarking information gathered by the committee indicates that the United States is serving a leadership role within the nanotechnology R&D communities but that the U.S. lead is facing significant and increasing international competition. Despite the lack of uniformity in countries' methods of calculating expenditures and allocating budgets, the committee compared U.S. public spending on R&D with spending by other governments and found that in general terms spending in Japan and spending across the European Union for nanoscale R&D are each comparable to the current annual U.S. investment of $1 billion in nanotechnology and nanoscience.

Country-by-country analyses of data on the number of papers published in leading scientific journals and on the number of patents awarded indicate significant growth worldwide in nanotechnology R&D and related intellectual property activity (see the section "Benchmarking Output: Indicators of Outcomes from Investment in Nanotechnology" in Chapter 2 for more detail). As a percentage of nanoscience and nanoengineering published papers, the fraction originating from the United States declined from 40 percent in the early 1990s to less than 30 percent in 2004, whereas U.S.-based entities continued to lead in the number of U.S. patents awarded.[9]

Currently, reliable data are not available that would allow linking technology transfer with confidence to specific NNI-related research programs, although the committee did discern positive trends in, for instance, patents awarded, venture capital activities, and the emergence of new small businesses (see the section "Technology Transfer" in Chapter 3). Looking at the economic impact of nanotechnology more broadly, as discussed in detail in Chapter 3, the committee concluded that it is too early to quantify the economic impact of nanotechnology. Neither have data been collected nor metrics developed that would enable a rigorous analysis of the economic impacts of nanoscale R&D. Moreover, as both an enabling and a disruptive technology, nanotechnology can be expected to have applications and effects that extend beyond a specific industry or market sector, leading to new products as well as improving already-available products. Yet it is clear that the promise of significant benefits in many areas of societal importance—in medicine, energy applications, national security, and so on—has led countries to invest billions of dollars globally in nanotechnology R&D.

NEXT STEPS—REALIZING THE PROMISE OF THE NNI

The federal investments in nanoscale R&D of the past several years are now beginning to bear fruit, providing a framework for continuing growth and achievement. NNI-related R&D, including cutting-edge basic research, is laying the groundwork for fundamental discoveries and innovation essential to the production of valuable and marketable new technologies, processes, and techniques. Full exploitation of nanotechnology, however, will require sustained commitments, consistent public and private support, and realistic expectations regarding returns on investment. To translate scientific excellence into economically viable technological products requires that policies and programs be in place that facilitate and also capitalize on the participation of both the public and the private sectors. Achieving and sustaining future advances will depend on productive partnerships among government, industry, and academia; new investments at the federal and state levels; and renewed commitments to both research and education. To enhance the prospects for continuing U.S. progress and leadership in nanoscale science and technology, the committee offers several recommendations based on findings developed in the course of its meetings and information gathered at its workshops.

Maintaining Support for the NNI

The committee found that the significant U.S. investment in the NNI to date has set the stage for ongoing valuable advances at the nanoscale by U.S. scientists and engineers over the next decade. Greater than the sum of its parts, the NNI is successfully establishing R&D programs with wider impact than could have been expected from separate agency funding without coordination. A multidisciplinary collaborative approach has enabled the NNI to advance basic research for the creation of foundational knowledge, support targeted applied research for high-impact applications, and establish new infrastructure for continued growth of interdisciplinary programs. Federal investments under the NNI are developing the investigative R&D tools—facilities and instruments that enable discovery and development—particularly unique, expensive, or large-scale tools beyond the means of a single organization. The NNI has also created interdisciplinary linkages that will be a lasting legacy of the initiative. In addition, the committee believes that federal agencies have been motivated by their participation in NNI activities to establish priorities, coordinate programs, and leverage resources to a degree that has proved very effective.

At a time of restrained R&D budgets, the committee stresses the importance of balancing federal support in pursuit of shorter-term research goals with longer-term R&D programs when budgets are being prioritized. Achieving a balanced program will require that federal support for basic nanoscale research not be compromised in favor of applied shorter-term technology work. Basic research and applied research are equally important, each with a different characteristic timescale within which benefits can be realized and goals reached. Two essential inputs to establishing balance in the NNI are the continued operation of the interagency coordination mechanisms and access to effective advice from members of the R&D community who have specific expertise to address technical areas and cross-disciplinary issues in nanoscale science and technology.

The committee notes that sustaining the capacity for U.S. science and technology advances into the future means not just providing financial support for NNI R&D but also ensuring a robust R&D infrastructure, broadly defined. Currently the NNI supports research that provides graduate students in the United States access to world-class education and research training opportunities, thereby contributing to the development of a workforce with skills for the 21st century. Throughout its study the committee heard of research from around the world that is important to U.S. efforts to meet the goals of the NNI, and it is widely recognized that in the United States visiting and domiciled foreign-born researchers and students are key contributors to all science and engineering fields. Their scientific knowledge and technical expertise contribute substantially to stimulating innovation, to this country's significant benefit. Continuing to attract the world's best students and researchers interested in nanotechnology will depend partly on how policies and the implementation of legal frameworks, such as immigration law and export control law, help or hinder international collaboration. The committee believes an important role of the NNI involves articulating to the NNI-participating federal agencies, to other relevant branches of the federal government, and to the U.S. Congress the importance of (1) maintaining the openness of the U.S. R&D enterprise to global partnerships and (2) ensuring the development of a high-quality U.S. science and technology workforce regardless of national origins. The U.S. visa system and the export control and licensing system can be supportive of, rather than barriers to, R&D, especially university-based and precompetitive research.

Recommendation. *In view of the NNI's evident progress toward developing a framework essential to maintaining and enhancing the nation's competitive position in nanoscale science and technology, the committee recommends that the federal government sustain investments in a manner that balances the pursuit of shorter-term goals with support for longer-term R&D and that ensures a robust supporting infrastructure,* *broadly defined. Supporting long-term research effectively will require making new funds available that do not come at the expense of much-needed ongoing investment in U.S. physical sciences and engineering research.*

Ensuring Access to Relevant Scientific Advice

The committee found that although the federal agencies each have internal mechanisms for soliciting and being guided by scientific advice, the NNI as a program does not have the benefit of access to an independent standing technical advisory panel with operational experience in research management and nanoscale R&D. Because of its size and scope, the NNI merits a dedicated and effective advisory panel well positioned to provide advice on (1) prioritizing support for short- and long-term research, (2) balancing the allocation of resources for large-scale centers and individual-investigator-led projects, and (3) giving expert opinions on the value of high-risk but high-pay-off research requiring interdisciplinary expertise.

The designation in 2004 of PCAST—the nation's preeminent committee of science advisors to the government—as the National Nanotechnology Advisory Panel was a welcome testament to the NNI's importance to the country. However, as discussed in more detail in Chapter 1, there is an ongoing national need for an independent panel of scientific and technical advisors whose experience includes, for instance, operational expertise specific to nanotechnology and nanoscience. Such an advisory panel would be available to provide advice to PCAST, NSET, and NNCO. The many advisory committees established across the federal government that operate under the Federal Advisory Committee Act provide multiple successful models for emulation in establishing this nanoscale-focused advisory resource.

Recommendation. *So that a source of independent expert advice on nanoscience and nanotechnology is readily available to the NSET Subcommittee, the NNCO, and PCAST, the committee recommends that the federal government establish an independent advisory panel with specific operational expertise in nanoscale science and engineering; management of research centers, facilities, and partnerships; and interdisciplinary collaboration to facilitate cutting-edge research on and effective and responsible development of nanotechnology.*

Satisfying the Need for More Data as a Basis for Prioritizing Investment and Measuring Impact

As is emphasized in Chapter 3, the committee found that U.S. federal investments in nanotechnology are not tracked and reported in a consistent way. Descriptions of funding requests, authorizations, budgets, and expenditures are neither uniform nor consistent across agencies. The dearth of data limits any analysis of the economic impact of the NNI or activity such as technology transfer. The committee recognizes that the budget preparation process within an agency is complex and differs widely from agency to agency. But as the complexity and the magnitude of the NNI grow, it is important that the nation have the ability to evaluate its investments in nanotechnology and to analyze how the return on those investments aligns with stated goals.

More consistent reporting across all agencies will lead to better determination of priorities for nanoscale-related funding. Properly constituted, an NNI advisory panel would be well positioned to oversee and advise on this process. The present PCA framework is a good one within which to conduct a comparative analysis of year-to-year budget requests and expenditures agency by agency, and PCA by PCA. For the larger federal agencies, further intra-agency breakdowns are naturally necessary.

Developing new indicators of and methodologies for assessing economic impact will have to be studied if future assessments are to be more quantitative rather than qualitative. The NSET Subcommittee co-chairs should make a priority of determining how to establish a foundation of data to aid policy and decision makers in future analyses. The methodology for any evaluation of economic impact might include, for example, best-effort evaluations of innovations in existing and new companies that have led to new products and new industrial processes. Although these efforts toward commercialization of nanotechnology are in their early stages, it is important to initiate now the development of indicators for these activities and, looking forward, to maintain databases on the relevant commercial activities, and on technology transfer from R&D into commercial application, over the life of the NNI.

Recommendation. *To build a capability for assessing the contribution of NNI investments to individual agencies' strategic goals and the broader goals of the NNI itself, the committee recommends that the federal agencies participating in the NNI, in consultation with the NNCO and the Office of Management and Budget, continue to develop and enhance means for consistent tracking and reporting of funds requested, authorized, and expended annually. The current set of PCAs provides an appropriate initial template for such tracking.*

Recommendation. *To establish a basis for assessing the NNI's economic impact over time, the committee recommends that, as an initial step, the NSET Subcommittee carry out or commission a study on the feasibility of developing metrics to quantify* *the return to the U.S. economy from the federal investment in nanotechnology R&D. The study should draw on the Department of Commerce's expertise in economic analysis and its existing ability to poll U.S. industry. Among the activities for which metrics should be developed and relevant data collected are technology transfer and commercial development of nanotechnology.*

Educating a 21st-Century Workforce

The committee found that the four existing NNI working groups, despite their considerable accomplishments, have not been able to bring a high level of coordination or management to the NNI goal of developing educational resources and a skilled workforce to support advances in nanotechnology. Representatives of corporations interviewed for this study indicated to the committee that workers with interdisciplinary skills and expertise are what companies involved in nanotechnology R&D are looking for. Satisfying these workforce needs will require a new approach to science and engineering education and training.

It is clear that nanotechnology is exciting K-12 students' interest in science, and this trend should be nurtured. Several workshops held under the auspices of the NNI have addressed the importance of incorporating new knowledge from nanoscale R&D into courses of study and workforce development. As new participants in the NNI, the Department of Education and the Department of Labor could help frame and prioritize related issues in and challenges posed for K-12 education and the nation's workforce. An education working group within the NSET Subcommittee could identify opportunities for agency and interagency activities and initiatives to strengthen the education of the 21st-century workforce. This new approach would complement ongoing work in education by science and technology agencies whose mission integrates educational objectives with research support, such as the National Science Foundation.

Recommendation. *Given that interest in nanotechnology presents a significant opportunity to stimulate renewed involvement in science and technology education and thereby strengthen the nation's workforce, the committee recommends that the NSET Subcommittee create a working group on education and the workforce that engages the Department of Education and the Department of Labor as active participants.*

Ensuring Responsible Development of Nanotechnologies—
Expanding Research on Environmental, Health, and Safety Effects

According to the NSET Subcommittee, the societal dimensions of the responsible development of nanotechnology encompass (1) research to characterize environmental, health, and safety (EHS) impacts of the development of nanotechnology and assessment of associated risks; (2) education-related activities such as development of materials for schools and undergraduate programs, technical training, and public outreach; and (3) research directed at identifying and quantifying the broad implications of nanotechnology for society, including social, economic, workforce, educational, ethical, and legal implications.[10]

The committee's analysis of responsible development focused on current EHS research (see the section "Environmental Health and Safety" and its subsection "The Current State of Published EHS Research" in Chapter 4 for details). The committee found that the results of EHS research to date and data on the EHS impacts of nanotechnology are inconclusive, and that risk assessment protocols have to be further developed and more research has to be done to assess the potential for EHS hazards from nanomaterials.

Although there is some evidence that engineered nanomaterials can have adverse effects on the health of laboratory animals, a lack of well-defined controls in experiments attempting to characterize nanomaterials and their effects and a lack of in vitro and in vivo studies contribute to the ambiguity of available data on EHS impacts of nanotechnology development. Obtaining valid EHS data will require an expanded research effort to support the important continuing dialog on these issues. Reproducible and well-characterized EHS data will inform the development of rigorous risk-based guidelines and best practices, but until that information becomes available, it is prudent to employ some precautionary measures to protect the health and safety of workers, the public, and the environment.

The committee notes that the NNI's NEHI working group has provided opportunities for exchange of information among agencies that support nanotechnology research and/or those responsible for regulation and guidelines related to nanoproducts and has helped to facilitate the identification, prioritization, and implementation of research and other activities required for the responsible development of nanotechnology.

Recommendation. To help ensure the responsible development of nanotechnology, the committee recommends that research on the environmental, health, and safety effects of nanotechnology be expanded. Assessing the effects of engineered nanomaterials on public health and the environment requires that the research conducted be well defined and reproducible and that effective methods be developed and applied to (1) estimate the exposure of humans, wildlife, and other ecological receptors to source material; (2) assess effects on human health and ecosystems of both occupational and environmental exposure; and (3) characterize, assess, and manage the risks associated with exposure.

Addressing the ethical and social impacts of nanotechnology will require an integrated approach involving scientists, engineers, social scientists, toxicologists, policymakers, and the public. The engagement and participation of the public are also necessary components of a national effort to ensure responsible development of nanotechnology.

Is Molecular Self-Assembly Feasible for Manufacturing?

Based on its examination of current manufacturing processes, the committee concluded that molecular self-assembly is feasible for the manufacture of simple materials and devices. However, for the manufacture of more sophisticated materials and devices, including complex objects produced in large quantities, it is unlikely that simple self-assembly processes will yield the desired results. The reason is that the probability of an error occurring at some point in the process will increase with the complexity of the system and the number of parts that must interoperate. In Chapter 5 the committee discusses lithography and nanobiotechnology as two areas relevant to so-called bottom-up or molecular manufacturing.

Biological systems, ranging in complexity from ribosomes, to viruses, to bacteria, to complex eukaryotic organisms, have been characterized as nature's perfect machinery. Demonstrations that biological systems can be engineered to operate outside a living cell and in alternate configurations suggest the possibility of a potential model for future manufacturing systems. However, it is difficult to reliably predict the attainable range of chemical reaction cycles, error rates, speed of operation, and thermodynamic efficiencies of such bottom-up manufacturing systems. Although theoretical thermodynamic efficiencies have been calculated for such systems, the committee did not learn of verifiable results of experimentation that would support reliable prediction of the feasibility of such systems for use in manufacturing. Experimentation leading to demonstrations supplying ground truth for abstract models is appropriate to better characterize the potential for use of bottom-up or molecular manufacturing systems that utilize processes more complex than self-assembly.

NOTES

1. Nanoscale Science, Engineering and Technology Subcommittee, Committee on Technology, National Science and Technology Council. 2005. The National Nanotechnology Initiative: Research and Development Leading to a Revolution in Technology and Industry. Supplement to the President's FY 2006 Budget Request. March. See the subsection "Federal Support for NNI R&D" in Chapter 1 for more information on the budget and the agencies involved.

2. Executive Order 13349 was signed on July 23, 2004, to designate PCAST to serve as the NNAP.

3. The subsection "Development of an Updated Strategic Plan" in Chapter 1 gives details on the genesis of these goals.

4. The PCAs are (1) fundamental nanoscale phenomena and processes; (2) nanomaterials; (3) nanoscale devices and systems; (4) instrumentation research, metrology, and standards for nanotechnology; (5) nanomanufacturing; (6) major research facilities and instrumentation acquisition; and (7) societal dimensions.

5. See the subsections "Establishment of Working Groups and Other Mechanisms for Coordination, Communication, and Outreach," "Solicitation of New Inter- and Intra-agency Collaborative Research," and "Investment in Centers and Networks for Multidisciplinary Nanoscale R&D" in Chapter 1 for details.

6. See http://www.nnin.org/, accessed June 2006.

7. See http://www.science.doe.gov/Sub/Newsroom/News_Releases/DOE-SC/2006/nano/index.htm, accessed June 2006.

8. M.C. Roco, NSET/NSF, presentation to this committee, June 27, 2005.

9. In 2003, the United States had 5,228 nanotechnology U.S. patents awarded, as compared to Japan (926), Germany (684), Canada (244), and France (183). U.S.-based entities accounted for about 67 percent of nanotechnology patents recorded in the U.S. Patent and Trademark Office database during the years 1976 to 2003.

10. Nanoscale Science, Engineering and Technology Subcommittee, Committee on Technology, National Science and Technology Council. 2005. The National Nanotechnology Initiative: Research and Development Leading to a Revolution in Technology and Industry. Supplement to the President's FY 2006 Budget Request. March.

1

A Review of the National Nanotechnology Initiative

In the mid-1990s, as better methods for the characterization, processing, and manipulation of matter at the nanoscale were being developed in research programs supported by the science and technology agencies of the federal government, these agencies began holding informal discussions on a common vision for what became known as nanotechnology (see Box 1-1 for a discussion of some definitions of nanotechnology). This interagency dialog culminated in the establishment in 2000 of the National Nanotechnology Initiative (NNI)—Box 1-2 details some of the history of the establishment of the initiative.

It is important to note at the outset that the initiative itself does not fund research. The NNI is a coordination mechanism for government agencies that support nanoscale research, such as the Department of Energy and the National Science Foundation, or that have a stake in the outcomes of nanoscale research, such as the Food and Drug Administration or the Department of Justice. Under the broad umbrella of the initiative, each participating agency invests in projects and programs in support of its own mission. The NNI itself also has a mission that can be summarized as expediting the discovery, development, and deployment of nanotechnology in order to achieve responsible and sustainable economic benefits, enhance the quality of life, and promote national security.[1] The initiative's primary coordination mechanism is the National Science and Technology Council's (NSTC's) Nanoscale Science, Engineering, and Technology (NSET) Subcommittee.[2] Through the operation of the NSET Subcommittee and the other subordinate structures of the NNI, the initiative addresses the general goals of supporting

BOX 1-1
What Is Nanotechnology?

Nanotechnology is not simply about small particles, materials, or products. It is not one type of technology with a defined use. Rather, nanotechnology is an enabling technology that promises to contribute at many frontiers of science and technology. For purposes of federal R&D, nanotechnology is defined by the National Nanotechnology Initiative as comprising the following three factors:[1]

1. Research and technology development at the atomic, molecular, or macromolecular levels, at a length scale of approximately 1 to 100 nanometers (a nanometer is one-billionth of a meter, too small to be seen with a conventional laboratory microscope);
2. Creation and use of structures, devices, and systems that have novel properties and functions because of their small and/or intermediate size, at the level of atoms and molecules;
3. Ability for atomic-scale control or manipulation.

The National Institutes of Health has further clarified the definition of nanotechnology, given that much of biomedical R&D involves work at the level of submicron features.[2,3] "Nano-medicine," for example, refers to highly specific medical intervention at the molecular scale for treating disease or repairing damaged tissues, such as bone, muscle, or nerve. It is at this size scale—about 100 nanometers or less—that biological molecules and structures inside living cells operate.

Research in nanotechnology is based on discoveries in physics and chemistry that have led to essential understanding of the physical and chemical properties of materials at the level of molecules or complexes of molecules, and thus to the ability to manipulate those properties. Researchers have characterized the parts of cells in vivid detail and now know a great deal about how intracellular structures operate, for example, but still have not been able to answer questions basic to understanding how to build "nano" structures or "nano" machines that are compatible with living tissues. In this and other areas of application, nanotechnology as an enabler of significant breakthroughs and benefits is still very much a young and developing endeavor.

---

[1]See http://nano.gov/html/facts/whatIsNano.html, accessed March 2006.
[2]See http://nihroadmap.nih.gov/nanomedicine/index.asp, accessed March 2006.
[3]National Science and Technology Council (NSTC). 2005. Nanobiotechnology: Report of the National Nanotechnology Initiative Workshop. Washington, D.C.: NSTC. August.

BOX 1-2
A Brief History of the National Nanotechnology Initiative

In September 1998, an ongoing interagency dialog on nanotechnology was formalized as the Interagency Working Group on Nanotechnology (IWGN). Established under the National Science and Technology Council (NSTC) of the Office of Science and Technology Policy, the IWGN developed a number of reports on a long-term vision for nanoscale R&D, on international benchmarking of nanotechnology, and on U.S. government investment in nanotechnology research and development (R&D).[1,2] In March 1999, IWGN representatives proposed a nanotechnology initiative with a budget of half a billion dollars for fiscal year (FY) 2001.[3] In January 2000, the National Nanotechnology Initiative (NNI) was formally established, and preparations were begun for a coordinated federal investment in nanoscale R&D.

In August 2000, as the NNI got underway, the NSTC established the Nanoscale Science, Engineering and Technology (NSET) Subcommittee to replace the IWGN. The NSET Subcommittee was tasked to implement the NNI by coordinating with federal agencies and R&D programs. At the time of this writing the NSET Subcommittee comprises representatives of over 20 federal departments and agencies along with officials from the White House Office of Science and Technology Policy and the White House Office of Management and Budget.

In January 2001, the National Nanotechnology Coordination Office (NNCO) was established to provide daily technical and administrative support to the NSET Subcommittee and to assist in multiagency planning and the preparation of budgets and program assessment documents. The NNCO was also tasked with assisting the NSET Subcommittee with the collection and dissemination of information on industry, state, and international nanoscale science and technology research, development, and commercialization activities.[4] The NNCO provides technical guidance and administrative support, organizes monthly NSET Subcommittee meetings, conducts workshops, and prepares information and reports, serving as a point of contact and helping to facilitate communication. Currently, these important operational functions are managed by a small group of scientific experts and technical staff.

---

[1]M.C. Roco, S. Williams, and P. Alivisatos, eds. 2000. Vision for Nanotechnology Research in the Next Decade. Nanotechnology Research Directions, IWGN Workshop Report. Kluwer Academic Publishers.

[2]R.W. Siegel, E. Hu, and M.C. Roco, eds. 1999. Nanostructure Science and Technology. Kluwer Academic Publishers.

[3]M.C. Roco. 2004. The U.S. National Nanotechnology Initiative after 3 years (2001-2003). Journal of Nanoparticle Research 6: 1010.

[4]National Research Council. 2002. Small Wonders, Endless Frontiers: A Review of the National Nanotechnology Initiative. Washington, D.C.: National Academy Press.

the missions of the participating agencies; ensuring continuing leadership by the United States in nanoscale science, engineering, and technology; and contributing to the nation's economic competitiveness.

CONTEXT FOR CURRENT OPERATION OF THE NNI

Management and Advisory Structure

In December 2003, the 21st Century Nanotechnology Research and Development Act[3] (NRDA) was signed into law, putting the NNI on a legislative footing that had been lacking. The legislation established the NNI's operating structures and also requested that the President establish and designate an advisory panel with a membership qualified to provide advice and information on nanotechnology research, development, demonstrations, education, technology transfer, commercial applications, and societal and ethical concerns.[4] Figure 1-1 shows the current organizational structure of the NNI.

The NRDA said that the President, in selecting or designating an advisory panel, might seek and give consideration to recommendations from the Congress, industry, the scientific community (including the National Academy of Sciences, scientific professional societies, and academia), the defense community, state and local governments, regional nanotechnology programs, and other appropriate organizations. According to the NRDA, the responsibilities of the advisory panel were to include assessing the following:

- Trends and developments in nanotechnology science and engineering;
- Progress made in implementing the NNI;
- Need for revision of the NNI;
- Balance among the components of the NNI, including funding levels for the program component areas;
- Whether the program component areas, priorities, and technical goals developed by the NSET Subcommittee were helping to maintain U.S. leadership in nanotechnology;
- Management, coordination, implementation, and activities of the NNI; and
- Whether societal, ethical, legal, environmental, and workforce concerns were being adequately addressed.

The NRDA also directed the National Nanotechnology Coordination Office (NNCO) to arrange with the National Research Council (NRC) for a triennial review of the NNI—of which this report is the first—and it asked that an NNI

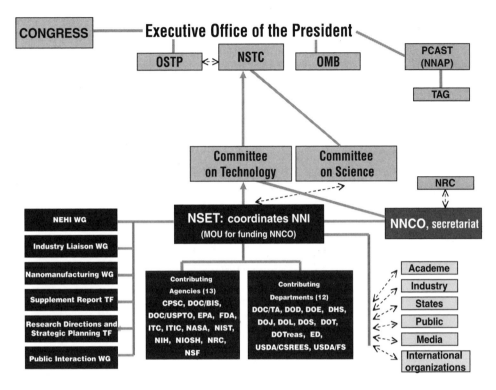

FIGURE 1-1 Organization of the NNI. Light shading, supervising organizations; dark shading, implementing organizations; PCAST, TAG, and NRC, organizations evaluating the NNI; dashed lines, lines of information exchange. For definitions of acronyms, see Appendix E. SOURCE: Courtesy of Mihail C. Roco, NSET/NSF.

strategic plan be developed, and then updated on a 3-year cycle, to guide the initiative's activities. It specified that the strategic plan should describe how the initiative would move R&D results out of the laboratory and into applications for the benefit of society; indicate the initiative's support for long-term funding for interdisciplinary research and development in nanotechnology; and outline the allocation of funding for interagency nanotechnology projects.

In response to the NRDA, in July 2004 President George W. Bush announced that the President's Committee of Advisors on Science and Technology (PCAST) would serve as the National Nanotechnology Advisory Panel (NNAP). PCAST provides broad science and technology policy advice to the President and has the expertise to address a wide range of technical, business, and policy issues. Because of its broad purview, PCAST created a nanotechnology technical advisory group

(TAG) of about 50 government and private sector scientists to assist it in the execution of its NNAP duties.

The first PCAST/NNAP report, released on May 18, 2005, reviewed the NNI after 5 years of operation.[5] The report focused on answering four questions: Where do we stand? Is this money well spent and the program well managed? Are we addressing societal concerns and potential risks? How can we do better? The PCAST/NNAP report made recommendations for strengthening NNI efforts in several areas:

- Improved technology transfer from the laboratory to the marketplace by communicating and establishing networks with U.S. industry;
- Increased coordination with and outreach to the states in support of nanotechnology R&D;
- Establishment of databases to improve the management of research results, publications, and patents resulting from researchers' use of NNI-supported facilities and instrumentation;
- Continued support for research on the effects of nanotechnology products to ensure protection of the public and the environment and establishment of regulatory standards and policies based on rational interpretation of science results, and not on perceived fears; and
- Inclusion in the NNI of the Departments of Education and Labor to improve the nation's science, technology, engineering, and mathematics education and training systems.

During the course of the present NRC study the Committee to Review the National Nanotechnology Initiative gave considerable thought to the effectiveness of the current NNI management and advisory structures outlined above. The committee's conclusions, based on its assessment of the overall effectiveness of the NNI in carrying out its coordination mission as described in the following sections, can be found at the end of this chapter in the section titled "Conclusions and Recommendations."

Federal Support for NNI R&D

Eleven NNI-participating agencies currently report investments in nanotechnology. They are the Department of Agriculture (USDA), Department of Defense (DOD), Department of Energy (DOE), Department of Homeland Security (DHS), Department of Justice (DOJ), Environmental Protection Agency (EPA), National Aeronautics and Space Administration (NASA), National Institute of Occupational Safety and Health (NIOSH), National Institute of Standards and Technology

TABLE 1-1 2006 Planned Agency Investments by Program Component Area (in $ millions)

	Fundamental Nanoscale Phenomena and Processes	Nanomaterials	Nanoscale Devices and Systems	Instrumentation Research, Metrology, and Standards for Nanotechnology	Nanomanufacturing	Major Research Facilities and Instrumentation Acquisition	Societal Dimensions	NNI Total[a]
NSF	95	75	54	12	24	24	60	344
DOD	35	83	99	3	2	6	2	230
DOE	48	33	5	11	0	109	1	207
HHS (NIH)	46	17	67	6	0	1	8	144
DOC (NIST)	5	1	2	39	19	8	1	75
NASA	4	17	10	0	1	0	0	32
USDA	1	2	6	0	1	0	1	11
EPA	<0.5	0	<0.5	0	0	0	4	5
HHS (NIOSH)	0	0	0	0	0	0	3	3
DOJ	0	0	0	0	0	0	2	2
DHS	0	0	1	0	0	0	0	1
TOTAL	234	228	244	71	47	148	82	1,054

[a]Totals may not add due to rounding.

SOURCE: Nanoscale Science, Engineering, and Technology Subcommittee, Committee on Technology, National Science and Technology Council. 2005. The National Nanotechnology Initiative: Research and Development Leading to a Revolution in Technology and Industry. Supplement to the President's FY 2006 Budget Request. March.

(NIST), National Institutes of Health (NIH), and National Science Foundation (NSF). In fiscal year (FY) 2005 the total investment made by these 11 agencies was about $1.1 billion—with DOD, DOE, NIH, NIST, and NSF contributing over 95 percent of the total NNI budget.[6] The President's R&D budget request for NNI for FY 2006 was $1.05 billion. For FY 2007 the request is $1.277 billion. Table 1-1 shows the FY 2006 planned agency budgets by program component area.[7] The committee notes that there is nanotechnology research being performed by some agencies that is not reported in this total.

The FY 2006 total federal science and technology R&D investment of $134.8 billion is a $2.2 billion or 1.7 percent increase over the FY 2005 amount, but it has been reported that 97 percent of this increase is for DOD weapons development and NASA next-generation space exploration vehicles.[8] Funding for all other R&D

programs increased marginally and actually fell 2 percent after adjusting for inflation. The total federal research investment (basic and applied), excluding development and R&D facilities, totaled $57.0 billion in FY 2006, an increase of $1.0 billion or 1.8 percent over the FY 2005 amount.

In the FY 2007 budget proposed by President Bush, programs in the physical sciences and engineering received a substantial funding increase as part of the American Competitiveness Initiative.[9] The three agencies benefiting the most from this increase are NSF, DOE's Office of Science, and NIST. The overall federal investment in science and technology R&D would increase to $136.9 billion in FY 2007, but the federal investment in basic and applied research would decline 3.3 percent to $54.8 billion. These numbers imply that the increases for the physical sciences will be more than offset by cuts in other agencies' research.

NNI ACCOMPLISHMENTS

In reviewing the NNI the committee investigated the various impacts the initiative has had, focusing, in particular, on the impact of NNI coordination—including the impacts on agency programs and priorities. The committee notes that it was clear early on that carrying out a comprehensive assessment of the science being funded by the NNI was beyond the means available to the study. The field of nanotechnology is so broad and involves so many disciplines that assessing the science output attributable to the NNI would be an enormously difficult task. A comprehensive study would require a thorough assessment of research programs across the 11 NNI-participating agencies, involving tremendously diverse fields spanning the physical and biomedical sciences. These difficulties notwithstanding, the committee did make some broad measurements of the value of the scientific endeavor under the NNI in its benchmarking assessment as reported in Chapter 2—for instance, by analyzing data on papers published and patents awarded. A workshop organized by the committee to obtain information on aspects of the science output of the NNI provided some perspectives of leading nanoscale science and technology researchers.[10] The strong consensus at that workshop, in the interviews held as part of this study with representatives of private industry, and in other materials submitted to the committee was that NNI-related R&D is world-class and in many instances world-leading, and that it is making invaluable contributions to the advancement of knowledge and innovation in the United States.

Development of an Updated Strategic Plan

The committee believes that coordination of nanoscale R&D programs across the federal government is the main purpose of the NNI, and also that provision of

TABLE 1-2 Distribution of Responsibilities Within the National Nanotechnology Initiative

Arm	Primary Office	Responsibilities
Science policy management	Executive Office of the President, Office of Science and Technology Policy, National Science and Technology Council, President's Council of Advisors on Science and Technology	Establishment of nanotechnology as a high priority for R&D; budget creation and allocation of funding to agencies; negotiation with Congress
Program management and coordination	Nanoscale Science, Engineering, and Technology (NSET) Subcommittee and member federal agencies	Coordination and development of strategic plan; provision of mechanisms for interagency communication and coordination
Communication, execution, and reporting	National Nanotechnology Coordination Office	Publication of reports on behalf of the NSET Subcommittee and the National Nanotechnology Initiative (NNI) for use by Congress, academia, industry, and the public; communication and outreach as public point of contact for the NNI

SOURCE: C. Teague, NNCO, presentation to this committee, August 25, 2005.

that coordination and the resultant deliverables are critical measures of the NNI's impact. In carrying out this review, the committee compiled information on NNI strategic planning and management that have involved broad participation by federal agencies and extensive coordination within each agency. The responsibilities for the management, coordination, and communication functions of the initiative are outlined in Table 1-2. The initiative's coordination has involved building strong partnerships across the government to leverage investments by government (state, regional, and international), industry (companies, trade associations, and international organizations), and scientific communities (universities, national laboratories, scientific societies, and professional organizations).

Released in December 2004, the updated strategic plan looks 5 to 10 years ahead to outline a vision of the NNI as working for "a future in which the ability to understand and control matter on the nanoscale leads to a revolution in technology and industry."[11] The strategic plan describes four goals of the NNI and the strategy by which those goals are to be achieved. The goals are these:

- Maintain a world-class research and development program aimed at realizing the full potential of nanotechnology.
- Facilitate transfer of new technologies into products for economic growth, jobs, and other public benefit.

- Develop educational resources, a skilled workforce, and the supporting infrastructure and tools to advance nanotechnology.
- Support responsible development of nanotechnology.

The strategic plan also outlines program component areas (PCAs) that were developed as a means to categorize and describe the many different investments in nanotechnology R&D made by the federal agencies that support research (see Table 1-1). The PCAs provide a framework that allows the NSET Subcommittee, Office of Science and Technology Policy, Office of Management and Budget, and Congress to be informed of NNI-related activities in a consistent fashion and that facilitates the management of investments in each PCA and the coordination and direction of activities within the participating agencies. The seven PCAs are as follows:

- *Fundamental nanoscale phenomena and processes.* Discovery and development of scientific and engineering principles relating to new structures, processes, and mechanisms at the nanoscale;
- *Nanomaterials.* Research involving the design and synthesis of nano-structured materials in a controlled and targeted manner;
- *Nanoscale devices and systems.* Research that applies science and engineering principles at the nanoscale to create new or improve existing devices and systems;
- *Instrumentation research, metrology, and standards for nanotechnology.* R&D involving the development of tools to characterize, measure, synthesize, and design materials, structures, devices, and systems at the nanoscale. R&D involving development of standards for nomenclature, materials, processing, testing, characterizing, and manufacturing;
- *Nanomanufacturing.* R&D enabling scaled-up, reliable, cost-effective manufacturing of nanoscale materials, devices, structures, and systems via top-down or bottom-up processes;
- *Major research facilities and instrumentation acquisition.* Establishment of user facilities and new development of instrumentation to improve and advance the research infrastructure; and
- *Societal dimensions.*[12] Research that addresses societal implications of nanotechnology, including risk assessment and communication, occupational health, public health, and the environment.

Having reviewed the 2004 strategic plan, the committee concluded that the articulation of the NNI's strategic goals and the development of the related PCAs are an important outcome of the NNI that has had a positive impact on the provision of federal support for the fields and disciplines involved in research and development at the nanoscale.

The PCA framework and the multidisciplinary collaboration it fosters have enabled a more coherent approach to achieving the NNI's goals than would have been possible otherwise. As part of the process of defining the PCAs, each agency assessed how it contributes to the seven areas listed above.[13,14] The committee learned that for many of the NNI-participating agencies, the strategic planning process and the identification of the seven PCAs have been important for engaging the interest and securing the support of various units within each agency. For instance, the committee was informed that at NSF, since the quality of NNI-related proposals is high, a proposal reviewed well by one unit but not awarded support owing to a lack of funds is now often shared with other units for consideration in other programs, based on the merit of the work. This approach has become more prevalent because of the knowledge NSF units have gained of programs at other NSF units, in part as a result of NNI-related activities.[15]

The committee is convinced that the development and implementation of the NNI strategic plan are key to the science impact that the NNI can be expected to have, which according to the general consensus referred to above is thought to be positive, substantive, and significant. In addition, the strategy has led to the NNI contributing to the education of the 21st-century R&D workforce, as well as addressing societal issues such as health effects and environmental impact. Not only has the establishment of a strategic plan for the NNI had a positive impact in itself, but it has also led to several programmatic impacts at the participating agencies and to the establishment of new structures as described below.

Establishment of Working Groups and Other Mechanisms for Coordination, Communication, and Outreach

In pursuit of NNI goals the initiative has been a catalyst for a significant increase in interagency communication and coordination spearheaded primarily by the NSET Subcommittee. The subcommittee meets monthly, and meeting attendance is reported to be excellent, numbering consistently between 40 and 60 people. In addition to the important work done by the NSET Subcommittee is its establishment of four interagency working groups to address specific cross-agency issues in the context of NNI goals and the seven NNI PCAs. They are the Nanotechnology Environmental and Health Implications (NEHI) Working Group; the Industry Liaison Working Group; the Nanomanufacturing Working Group; and the Nanotechnology Public Interaction Working Group (see Figure 1-1).

The flexible structure of the working groups and focused discussions by participants help to promote effective interagency communication, coordination, and joint program development and enable the NSET Subcommittee to efficiently address societal issues by giving it ready access to regulatory experts and health professionals in various agencies.

The NEHI Working Group was formed during FY 2005 to facilitate coordination within and between agencies' environmental, health, and safety research programs relating to nanotechnology. It provides for exchange of information among agencies that support nanotechnology research and those responsible for regulations and guidelines related to nanoproducts (defined as engineered nanoscale materials, nanostructured materials or nanotechnology-based devices, and their byproducts); facilitates the identification, prioritization, and implementation of research and other activities required for responsible R&D on, and utilization and oversight of, nanotechnology, including research methods for life cycle analysis; and promotes communication of information related to research on environmental and health implications of nanotechnology to government agencies and nongovernment parties.

The Industry Liaison Working Group collaborates with representatives of the semiconductor, chemical, aerospace, biotechnology, and automotive industries to establish communication with the NNI-participating agencies, to provide industry with information on NNI's R&D activities, and to give industry an opportunity to offer suggestions on how the NNI might best support precompetitive R&D that meets industry needs. The Nanomanufacturing Working Group, which involves primarily NSF, DOD, and NIST, coordinates activities related to reliable, scaled-up manufacture of nanoscale materials, components, and products. The Nanotechnology Public Interaction Working Group was established to develop approaches by which the NNI can communicate more effectively with the public.

A separate effort toward broadening outreach involves the Global Issues in Nanotechnology Working Group, led by the State Department, which was established to engage additional federal agencies with international interests, such as the United States Trade Representative and the Bureau of Industry and Security at the Department of Commerce. It is to provide input on and coordinate U.S. international activities on nanotechnology, monitor international programs, and identify opportunities for international coordination and communication. Currently, this working group is in communication with U.S. delegates to and representatives of the Organisation for Economic Co-Operation and Development, the Asia-Pacific Economic Cooperation, the Wassenaar Arrangement,[16] and the President's Export Council's Subcommittee on Export Administration.

In another NNI outreach effort and in pursuit of the NNI's second goal of facilitating the transfer of new technologies into products for economic growth, jobs, and other public benefit, the NSET Subcommittee has established the Consultative Board for Advancing Nanotechnology (CBAN), which is charged with promoting a dialog on NNI-related research programs and industry needs relating to nanotechnology. CBAN has been working with the semiconductor, electronics, and chemical industries and plans to expand activities with other industry sectors. For example, in March 2004, under the auspices of the NNI, the Council for Chemical Research and the Chemical Industry Vision 2020 (ChI) formed a partnership to engage in activities involving joint planning and support of collaborative activities in key R&D areas, identifying and promoting new R&D for exploratory areas, and expanding nanotechnology R&D. One of the established NNI-ChI CBAN working groups is addressing environmental safety and health issues for nanotechnology.[17]

The NSET Subcommittee has utilized the Small Business Innovation Research program and the Small Business Technology Transfer program to support early-stage nanotechnology developments and to accelerate the transfer of newly developed nanotechnologies to practical commercial applications and public use. In addition, in November 2003, NSF and the Semiconductor Research Corporation (SRC), one of the Semiconductor Industry Association's affiliates, signed a statement of principles, "Silicon Nanoelectronics and Beyond," that outlines university research for future technologies at the nanoscale level.[18]

Having seen evidence of positive impacts of their efforts to date, the committee believes that the working groups and other outreach and coordination efforts stimulated by and established under the NNI have made a considerable contribution to coordination of R&D efforts in pursuit of realizing the full potential of nanotechnology.

Solicitation of New Inter- and Intra-agency Collaborative Research

A significant impact of the NNI has been the development of new collaborations across agencies and between different units within agencies that are conducting R&D relevant to the broad goals articulated by the NNI, as signified by announcements on the Web for programs such as the following:[19]

- Nanotechnology Research Grants Investigating Environmental and Human Health Effects of Manufactured Nanomaterials (2004), a program organized by the EPA, NSF's Engineering Directorate, NIOSH, the Centers for Disease Control and Prevention (CDC), and the Department of Health and Human Services (HHS), that sought proposals for investigating the potential implications of nanotechnology and manufactured nanomaterials for human health and the environment. Research areas included toxicology; fate, transport, and transformation; and exposure of humans and other species in natural ecosystems to nanomaterials.

- The NIH's National Cancer Institute and NSF awarded training grants for nanobiotechnology intended to facilitate greater diversity in the globally engaged science and engineering workforce by establishing integrative training environments for U.S. science and engineering doctoral students to focus on interdisciplinary nanoscience and technology research with applications to cancer.
- Interagency Opportunities in Metabolic Engineering, a program involving NSF, DOE, DOD, DOC, USDA, NIH, EPA, and NASA in a collaborative effort to provide an opportunity for an interagency granting activity in the area of metabolic engineering through in-kind support such as equipment, laboratory space, personnel time, and materials.
- The Nanotechnology Characterization Laboratory, an effort aimed at performing preclinical efficacy and toxicity testing of nanoparticles, with the National Cancer Institute as the lead agency, in strong collaboration with NIST and the Food and Drug Administration (FDA).
- The National Toxicology Program (NTP), a collaboration of the National Institute of Environmental Health Sciences of the NIH, the National Institute for Occupational Safety and Health/Centers for Disease Control and Prevention, and the National Center for Toxicological Research of the FDA. Under the NTP's broad-based research program to address potential human health hazards from unintentional exposure associated with the manufacture and use of new chemicals, an effort has been initiated to investigate the toxicology of nanoscale materials of current or projected commercial importance.
- Collaborations by the Naval Research Laboratory and NASA's Ames Research Center to develop single-molecule detection of trace levels of explosives.[20]

The NNI is also promoting intra-agency programs that cross disciplinary boundaries. Through the Interdisciplinary Training for Undergraduates in Biological and Mathematical Sciences program, the NSF's Directorate for Biological Sciences, in a joint effort with its Education and Human Resources and Mathematical and Physical Sciences directorates, is enhancing undergraduate education and training at the intersection of the biological and mathematical sciences, to better prepare undergraduate biology or mathematics students to pursue graduate study and careers in fields that integrate the mathematical and biological sciences. The NIH's Emerging Technologies for the Study of Reproductive Neuroendocrinology program involves the National Institute of Child Health and Human Development and the National Institute of Neurological Disorders and Stroke in an effort to stimulate the development of new technologies, including nanotechnology, to address issues in neuroendocrine control of the reproductive function.

Investment in Centers and Networks for Multidisciplinary Nanoscale R&D

The committee believes that a critically important impact of the NNI has been the focused investment by the NNI-participating agencies in the establishment and development of multidisciplinary research and education centers devoted to nanoscience and nanotechnology. Many such centers are designated as user facilities available to researchers from academia and the private sector, and to scientists at the national laboratories. Featuring physical facilities, equipment, instrumentation, technical expertise, and necessary operating personnel, the centers bring together researchers with a wide range of expertise in an array of disciplines. User facilities are powerful and efficient vehicles for broadening access to the scientific and technical resources currently funded by federal support from NNI-participating agencies. They are particularly important to the nanoscale science and technology community owing to the equipment-intensive nature of much of the characterization and processing of nanomaterials.

An illustrative list of centers is provided in Box 1-3. A few specific agency center activities, described below, are but some examples of how the NNI has affected the infrastructure for R&D in the United States. A recent survey by Asia Nano Forum, presented at the Global Nanotechnology Network (GNN) workshop in

---

BOX 1-3
Examples of Some NNI-related Centers with Support from DOD, DOE, NASA, NIOSH, NIST, and NSF

The following list illustrates the disciplinary and geographic diversity of the NNI-related centers supported by various federal departments and agencies at the time of this writing and is not intended to be complete or final.

DOD
- Institute for Soldier Nanotechnologies—Massachusetts Institute of Technology
- Center for Nanoscience Innovation for Defense—University of California Santa Barbara
- Institute for Nanoscience, Naval Research Laboratory

DOE Nanoscale Science Research Centers
- Center for Nanophase Materials Sciences, Oak Ridge National Laboratory
- Center for Functional Nanomaterials, Brookhaven National Laboratory
- Center for Integrated Nanotechnologies, Sandia National Laboratories
- Center for Nanoscale Materials, Argonne National Laboratory
- Molecular Foundry, Lawrence Berkeley National Laboratory

continued

BOX 1-3 Continued

NASA
- Institute for Cell Mimetic Space Exploration—University of California Los Angeles, Arizona State University, California Institute of Technology, University of California Irvine
- Institute for Intelligent Bio-Nanomaterials & Structures for Aerospace Vehicles—Texas A&M University, University of Texas at Arlington, University of Houston, Texas Southern University, Rice University, Prairie View A&M University
- Bio-Inspection, Design and Processing of Multi-functional Nanocomposites—Princeton University
- Institute for Nanoelectronics and Computing—Purdue University, Northwestern University, Cornell University, University of Florida, University of California San Diego, Yale University, Texas A&M University

NIOSH
- Center of Excellence in Nanotechnology Research

NIST User Centers
- Advanced Measurement Laboratory
- NIST Center for Neutron Research
- National Nanomanufacturing and Nanometrology Facility

NSF (NSEC, Nanoscale Science and Engineering Center)
- Center for Nanoscale Systems, Nanoscale Science and Engineering Center (NSEC)—Cornell University, Harvard University, Massachusetts Institute of Technology, University of California Santa Barbara, Delft University, University of Basel, University of Tokyo
- Center for Nanoscience in Biological & Environmental Engineering—Rice University, University of Texas
- Integrated Nanopatterning and Detection (NSEC)—Northwestern University, University of Chicago, University of Illinois at Urbana-Champaign, Harold Washington College
- Electron Transport in Molecular Nanostructures (NSEC)—Columbia University
- Nanoscale Systems and Their Device Applications (NSEC)—Harvard University, MIT, University of California Santa Barbara, Delft University of Technology, University of Basel, University of Tokyo
- Directed Assembly of Nanostructures (NSEC)—Rensselaer Polytechnic Institute, University of Illinois at Urbana-Champaign
- Nanobiotechnology, Science and Technology Center—Cornell University, Columbia University, Harvard University, Northwestern University, Rensselaer Polytechnic Institute, Rice University
- Extreme Ultraviolet Science and Technology—Colorado State University, University of California Berkeley, University of Colorado Boulder
- Center for Scalable and Integrated Nano-Manufacturing (NSEC)—UCLA, University of California Berkeley, Stanford University, University of California San Diego, University of North Carolina at Charlotte

- Center for Chemical-Electrical-Mechanical Manufacturing Systems (NSEC)—University of Illinois at Urbana-Champaign, California Institute of Technology, North Carolina Agricultural and Technological State University
- Templated Synthesis & Assembly at the Nanoscale—University of Wisconsin-Madison
- Molecular Function at NanoBio Interface—University of Pennsylvania, Drexel University
- High-Rate Nanomanufacturing—Northeastern University, University of Massachusetts Lowell, University of New Hampshire, Michigan State University
- Affordable Nanoengineering of Polymer Biomedical Devices—Ohio State University, University of California Berkeley, Northeastern University, University of Pennsylvania, Stanford University, University of Wisconsin-Madison
- Integrated Nanomechanical Systems—University of California Berkeley, Caltech, Stanford University, University of California Merced
- Probing the Nanoscale—Stanford University
- Learning & Teaching in Nano S&E—Northwestern University, Purdue University, University of Michigan, University of Illinois at Chicago, University of Illinois at Urbana-Champaign

NSF National Nanofabrication Infrastructure Network (NNIN)
- Cornell University, Cornell Nanoscale Science and Fabrication Facility
- Howard University, Keck Center for the Design of Nanoscale Materials for Molecular Recognition
- Pennsylvania State University, Nanofabrication Facility
- Stanford University, Stanford NanoFabrication Facility
- University of California Santa Barbara, Nanotech Fabrication Facility
- Georgia Institute of Technology, Microelectronics Research Laboratory
- Harvard University, Center for Imaging and Mesoscale Systems
- North Carolina State University, Triangle National Lithography Center
- University of Michigan, Solid State Electronics Laboratory
- University of Minnesota, Minnesota Nanotechnology Cluster
- University of New Mexico, Nanoscience at the University of New Mexico
- University of Texas at Austin, Microelectronics Research Center
- University of Washington, Center for Nanotechnology

NSF's Network for Computational Nanotechnology (NCN) for Nanoelectronics, Nanoelectromechanics, Nanobioelectronics
- Purdue University, University of Illinois, Stanford University, University of Florida, University of Texas El Paso, Northwestern University, Morgan State University

SOURCE: National Science and Technology Council (NSTC). 2004. The National Nanotechnology Initiative Strategic Plan. Washington, D.C.: NSTC. December. See also http://nano.gov/html/centers/nnicenters.html, accessed March 2006; also, Nanoscale Science, Engineering, and Technology Subcommittee, Committee on Technology, National Science and Technology Council, 2005, Research and Development Leading to a Revolution in Technology and Industry, Supplement to the President's FY 2006 Budget Request, March.

May 2005, indicates that the United States is among the world leaders in terms of funding for these infrastructure elements today.[21] According to the NNI, the budget requested for major research facilities and instrumentation acquisition in FY 2006 was $148 million, accounting for 14 percent of the budget.[22]

Department of Defense

The research mission of MIT's Institute for Soldier Nanotechnologies is to use nanotechnology to improve the survival of soldiers. The ultimate goal is to create a 21st-century battle suit that combines high-tech capabilities with light weight and comfort. Established in 2002, the institute is funded at $50 million for 5 years. The DOD-supported Center for Nanoscience Innovation in Defense, at the University of California, Santa Barbara, was created to facilitate the rapid transition of research innovation in the nanosciences into applications for the defense sector. It was established in 2002 and funded at $20 million for 3 years.

The Naval Research Laboratory's Institute for Nanoscience conducts interdisciplinary research at the intersections of the fields of materials, electronics, and biology in the nanometer size domain. The institute exploits the broad multidisciplinary character of the Naval Research Laboratory, bringing together scientists with disparate training and backgrounds to address common goals at the intersection of their respective fields at this length scale. The objective of the institute's programs is to provide the Navy and the DOD with scientific leadership in this complex, emerging area and to identify opportunities for advances in future defense technology.

Department of Energy

Five nanoscale science research centers (NSRCs) are under development by DOE and will be collocated with existing major facilities at DOE laboratories across the country. Upon completion, the NSRCs will be operated as user facilities that are accessible to all researchers on a merit-reviewed basis. The construction budget is about $60 million to $80 million per center, and the annual operational budget is about $20 million per center.

- The Center for Nanophase Materials Sciences, based at the Oak Ridge National Laboratory and the first of the DOE's NSRCs, includes a nanofabrication research laboratory with clean rooms and an area designated for electron-beam imaging with low levels of electromagnetic interference and vibration. The center is co-located with the new Spallation Neutron Source.

- The Center for Functional Nanomaterials, based at the Brookhaven National Laboratory, will focus on characterization of the chemical and physical response of nanomaterials as a basis for making functional materials such as sensors, activators, and energy-conversion devices.
- The Center for Integrated Nanotechnologies, involving Los Alamos National Laboratory and Sandia National Laboratories, will concentrate on nanophotonics and nanoelectronics, complex functional nanomaterials, nanomechanics, and nanoscale/bio/microscale interfaces.
- The Center for Nanoscale Materials, based at the Argonne National Laboratory, will focus on research in advanced magnetic materials, complex oxides, nanophotonics, and bioinorganic hybrids.
- The Molecular Foundry, at the Lawrence Berkeley National Laboratory, will use existing LBNL facilities such as the Advanced Light Source, the National Center for Electron Microscopy, and the National Energy Research Scientific Computing Center.

National Institute of Standards and Technology

NIST's National Nanomanufacturing and Nanometrology Facility supports the development of new infrastructural metrology and standards for U.S. nanotechnology efforts through centralized access to NIST's unique nanometrology and nanofabrication resources, including the facilities of the Advanced Measurement Laboratory and NIST's nanometrology experts at the Advanced Measurement Laboratory. It was started in 2005 with a $10 million budget. The NIST Center for Neutron Research is part of the Materials Science and Engineering Laboratory at NIST. Its activities are focused on provision of neutron measurement capabilities to researchers in the United States. It is a national center for research using thermal and cold neutrons, offering advanced measurement capabilities for use by all qualified applicants.[23]

National Science Foundation

The NSF's National Nanotechnology Infrastructure Network (NNIN) comprises facilities at 13 partner universities aimed at providing fabrication and characterization facilities, instrumentation, and expertise. These facilities either are subsidized or the full cost is recovered, and they are accessible through merit review. The NNIN was started in 2004, with more than $28 million allocated for the 5-year effort.

The NSF's Network for Computational Nanotechnology, started in 2002, includes seven universities that together support computational research, as well as education and modeling and simulation tools that can be accessed via the Web.

Announced in October 2005, the NSF's Nanoscale Informal Science Education Network award will support a national network of science museums, providing informal educational activities for schoolchildren as well as adults. Two centers for nanotechnology in society are being created through NSF funding and, through a network of social scientists, economists, and nanotechnology researchers, will formulate a long-term vision for addressing societal, ethical, environmental, and education concerns; involve partners or affiliates to collaborate on topics related to responsible nanotechnology; formulate plans to involve a wide range of stakeholders; and develop a clearinghouse for information on communicating about nanoscience and nanotechnology and engaging the public in meaningful dialog.[24]

EDUCATION, WORKFORCE, AND PUBLIC UNDERSTANDING

During the course of this study the committee heard from several sources, and indeed it is the experience of many educators on the committee, that NNI-related science and technology R&D and the strong federal support for discovery-based research and interdisciplinary collaborations at university centers are attracting and exciting students. For example, new research opportunities are drawing the attention of students to research at the interface of the physical and biomedical sciences, a direct benefit of collaborative federal funding by agencies such as NIH, NSF, and DOE.

While nanotechnology holds much promise for attracting students to the nation's research universities, it is troubling that math and science indicators at the K-12 level have been showing a steady decline in overall U.S. student performance.[25,26] Also, the number of U.S.-born and U.S.-educated students advancing into the science, technology, engineering, and mathematics (STEM) track is at an all-time low.[27] These trends continue despite a significant emphasis on teaching by federal research granting organizations such as NSF whose centers are serving important roles in this regard, and despite educational programs funded for K-12 students, college and graduate students, and general public understanding. Stronger STEM programs in K-12 education could leverage state initiatives, reach out to university education departments to train new teachers, and involve teachers' professional organizations (such as the National Council of Teachers of Mathematics and the Mathematical Association of America) for continuing education and certification. Recommendations for such changes were recently made in the National Research Council report *Rising Above the Gathering Storm: Energizing and Employing America for a Brighter Economic Future.*[28]

In addition to educating students, sharing the discoveries of science with a broader audience is an important responsibility of the science and technology community. Beyond efforts to impact K-16 education, understanding by and engagement of the public are important objectives that the science community must address, given that such understanding is basic to the public's trust in and support for nanotechnology R&D, on the one hand, and to the public's excitement about scientific exploration and discovery in general, on the other.

Science and engineering are not conducted in a vacuum. University education, including participation in the research conducted at universities, fosters the next generation of scientific thinkers. Industry R&D enables new products with better functionality, leading to manufacturing and jobs. Government leadership advances the best interests of the nation, maintaining an infrastructure for S&T excellence, stimulating industrial innovation, protecting the environment, improving health, and ensuring national security. And the general public, who are the catalyst for and beneficiaries of government's successes, must be kept informed.

Science in the media needs to reflect the challenges and opportunities that drive the scientific and technological infrastructure supported by federal funds and private investments. Many organizations, including the National Academies, have increased their public outreach activities with greater coverage on public radio and open access to their publications. With greater online access, NSF and DOE media Web sites have also increased their coverage with exciting news releases and featured stories. For example, it is worth noting that the NSF site on nanotechnology captures the imagination of many with news, discoveries, and images.[29,30] The committee believes that the public's curiosity about nanotechnology could be leveraged more effectively to build public support for the federal support of R&D in the physical and biomedical sciences, as well as attract new talent into U.S. undergraduate and graduate education.

CONCLUSIONS AND RECOMMENDATIONS

Revisiting the NNI's first three goals (see the subsection "Development of an Updated Strategic Plan" above in this chapter) provides a useful framework for summarizing the committee's conclusions about the impact of the NNI. The issue in the fourth goal, responsible development, is dealt with separately in this report in Chapter 4, in the context of the committee's separate task to consider that particular issue.

Goal 1: Maintain a World-Class Research and Development Program Aimed at Realizing the Full Potential of Nanotechnology

The committee notes that federal R&D programs are intended to advance the boundaries of knowledge and develop technologies that address government and national needs. To accomplish the vision of the NNI, a coordinated federal investment has been developed at the frontiers and intersections of many disciplines, including biology, chemistry, engineering, materials, and physics. Activities aimed at making progress toward the NNI's first goal include support for basic or knowledge-inspired research, and development of technology. Application areas of interest to both government and industry include the environment, health, medicine, energy, information technology, defense, transportation, and agriculture and food systems. NNI activities have produced significant advances in these and other application areas and are progressing from fundamental discovery to technological applications and commercialization.

The committee concluded that development of the goals articulated in the NNI's strategic plan and establishment of the related PCAs are an important outcome of the NNI that has had a positive impact on allocation of federal support to the fields and disciplines that make up nanotechnology. In addition, the committee is convinced that the successful coordination driven by the NSET Subcommittee and the coordination framework it has established are at the heart of the NNI's advances toward achievement of its first goal. The NNI is successfully coordinating nanoscale R&D efforts and interests across the government as the federal agencies supporting nanoscale research move toward a broadly common vision of federal investment in nanotechnology and nanoscience. The working groups and other outreach and coordination efforts developed under the initiative have contributed considerably to the development of new collaborations between agencies and between different units within agencies, all in pursuit of realizing the full potential of nanotechnology in the context of the NNI PCAs.

Research supported by NNI-participating agencies includes cutting-edge basic research leading to fundamental discoveries as a basis for producing valuable and marketable technologies, processes, and techniques. Federal investments under the NNI are developing the tools of science—facilities and instruments that enable discovery and development—particularly unique, expensive, or large-scale tools beyond the means of a single organization. The committee is convinced that the significant U.S. investment in the NNI to date and the resultant research progress have set the stage for even more valuable advances at the nanoscale by U.S. scientists and engineers in the next decade. The multidisciplinary collaborative approach fostered by the NNI has enabled advances in basic research for the creation of foundational knowledge, targeted applied research for high-impact applications, and established infrastructure for access to facilities, equipment, and instrumentation. The NNI has also created interdisciplinary linkages that otherwise are likely not to have formed. These new interconnections between fields and between individual scientists and engineers from a diverse range of fields will be a lasting legacy of the initiative.

At a time of restrained R&D budgets, the committee stresses the importance of balancing federal support in pursuit of shorter-term research goals with longer-term R&D programs when budgets are being prioritized. Achieving a balanced program will require that federal support for basic nanoscale research not be compromised in favor of applied shorter-term technology work. Basic research and applied research are equally important, each with a different characteristic timescale within which benefits can be realized and goals reached. Two essential inputs to establishing balance in the NNI are the continued operation of the interagency coordination mechanisms and access to effective advice from members of the R&D community who have specific expertise to address technical areas and cross-disciplinary issues in nanoscale science and technology.

The committee notes that sustaining the capacity for U.S. science and technology advances into the future means not just providing financial support for NNI R&D but also ensuring a robust R&D infrastructure, broadly defined. Currently the NNI supports research that provides graduate students in the United States access to world-class education and research training opportunities, thereby contributing to the development of a workforce with skills for the 21st century. Throughout its study the committee heard of research from around the world that is important to U.S. efforts to meet the goals of the NNI, and it is widely recognized that in the United States visiting and domiciled foreign-born researchers and students are key contributors to all science and engineering fields. Their scientific knowledge and technical expertise contribute substantially to stimulating innovation, to this country's significant benefit. Continuing to attract the world's best students and researchers interested in nanotechnology will depend partly on how policies and the implementation of legal frameworks, such as immigration law and export control law, help or hinder international collaboration. The committee believes an important role of the NNI involves articulating to the NNI-participating federal agencies, to other relevant branches of the federal government, and to the U.S. Congress the importance of (1) maintaining the openness of the U.S. R&D enterprise to global partnerships and (2) ensuring the development of a high-quality U.S. science and technology workforce regardless of national origins. The U.S. visa system and the export control and licensing system can be supportive of, rather than barriers to, R&D, especially university-based and precompetitive research.

In addition, the committee believes that federal agencies are motivated by their participation in NNI activities to establish priorities, coordinate programs, and leverage resources. The level of interagency collaborations has proved very effective. It deserves continuing strong support, and so the committee offers the following recommendation:

Recommendation. In view of the NNI's evident progress toward developing a framework essential to maintaining and enhancing the nation's competitive position in nanoscale science and technology, the committee recommends that the federal government sustain investments in a manner that balances the pursuit of shorter-term goals with support for longer-term R&D and that ensures a robust supporting infrastructure, broadly defined. Supporting long-term research effectively will require making new funds available that do not come at the expense of much-needed ongoing investment in U.S. physical sciences and engineering research.

Assessing the value to the nation's ongoing investments in NNI-related science, engineering, and technology will require that high-quality information and data be collected and made publicly available each year, and also that a baseline of information and data be established against which to assess the impacts of the federal investment in the NNI and thereby determine if NNI and national goals are being met. The committee acknowledges the challenges inherent in collecting, organizing, and tracking such data across agencies and notes the OMB's efforts to improve agencies' reporting of data on NNI-related research support. However, the committee is convinced that there is room for improvement in the reporting mechanisms so as to ensure improved transparency and confidence in the numbers. Efforts toward a coordinated system of consistent tracking and reporting should involve each NNI-participating agency equally and should include intra-agency actions as well.

Recommendation. To build a capability for assessing the contribution of NNI investments to individual agencies' strategic goals and the broader goals of the NNI itself, the committee recommends that the federal agencies participating in the NNI, in consultation with the NNCO and the Office of Management and Budget, continue to develop and enhance means for consistent reporting and tracking of funds requested, authorized, and expended annually. The current set of PCAs provides an appropriate initial template for such tracking.

Goal 2: Facilitate Transfer of New Technologies into Products for Economic Growth, Jobs, and Other Public Benefit

To achieve the full benefit of the results of NNI-funded R&D requires the transitioning of ideas into products. Technology transfer can occur via various pathways, including hiring of recent graduates and licensing of intellectual property resulting from federally funded research. A primary aspect of all technology transfer activities is interaction among those who are performing R&D and those who manufacture and sell goods and services. While NNI-stimulated interaction with industry has been encouraging, the committee welcomes NNI plans to further explore how to facilitate successful commercialization of nanotechnology. These issues are discussed in Chapter 3 on the economic impact of nanotechnology, which includes a recommendation to address the need for collecting data on and developing means to measure the transfer of technology from research to the marketplace, as well as the commercial development of nanotechnology.

Goal 3: Develop Educational Resources, a Skilled Workforce, and the Supporting Infrastructure and Tools to Advance Nanotechnology

A well-educated and skilled workforce, and a supporting infrastructure of instrumentation, equipment, and facilities, are essential to progress in developing nanotechnology. The committee believes that the NNI's progress on these deliverables has been good to date, but it believes that more attention is needed to education.

The federal government maintains a suite of user facilities that support nanoscale R&D, including, for example, the high-intensity X-ray and neutron source facilities operated by DOE, NSF, and NIST. A role of the NNI is to continue to develop infrastructure that specifically addresses the specialized needs of the nanotechnology research community, and federal support can make these state-of-the-art research capabilities accessible to researchers based on merit review.

Nanoscale science, engineering, and technology education can help to (1) produce the next generation of researchers and innovators, (2) provide the 21st-century workforce with the math and science education and technological skills it will need to succeed, and (3) inform decision makers in an increasingly technology-driven society. The committee heard from its interviews with representatives of corporations during this study that workers with interdisciplinary skills and background are what companies with R&D programs in nanotechnology are looking for. Satisfying the growing demand for a highly skilled workforce will require a new approach to science and technology education and training. In this regard, the committee notes that while the four existing NNI working groups have accomplished much, there has not been a similar level of coordination or management brought to the NNI goal of developing educational resources and a skilled workforce. It is abundantly clear that "nano" is exciting K-12 students' interest in science, and this trend should be nurtured. Several NNI workshops have addressed the need to coordinate nanoscale R&D with efforts to strengthen education and workforce development.

As new participants in the NNI, the Department of Education and the Department of Labor could help to frame and prioritize the main issues that nanoscale R&D poses for K-12 education and the nation's workforce. Involvement at the state and local levels could also help to ensure that national policy is flexible enough to accommodate local student needs, enhance teacher training, and encourage the public's participation in addressing issues related to science education and nanotechnology. This new approach would complement ongoing educational work by S&T agencies whose mission integrates educational objectives with research support, like the National Science Foundation.

In this regard, the committee offers the following recommendation:

Recommendation. *Given that interest in nanotechnology presents a significant opportunity to stimulate renewed involvement in science and technology education and thereby strengthen the nation's workforce, the committee recommends that the NSET Subcommittee create a working group on education and the workforce that engages the Department of Education and the Department of Labor as active participants.*

The committee believes that an educational working group within the NSET Subcommittee could consider the opportunities for agency and interagency initiatives to:

- Support the education of the 21st-century workforce;
- Encourage U.S. students to undertake graduate studies that include course work in nanoscale science and technology and continue on to work at U.S. scientific institutions;
- Stimulate dialog on undergraduate interdisciplinary education and the introduction of nanotechnology into current disciplinary curricula;
- Broker a national dialog involving the nanotechnology centers and facilities that are engaged in educational programs on each center's strengths and on regional needs and thereby enable a sharing of experiences;
- Leverage the public's interest in nanotechnology and broaden people's understanding, furthering the objective of encouraging minorities and women to take up careers as scientists and engineers;
- Encourage a dialog with the public and policymakers, in partnership with the working group on public engagement, on nanoscale science, technology, and medicine and their economic potential and societal impacts; and
- Initiate state and regional dialogs on nanoscale science and engineering education at precollege levels, engaging education professionals and community groups to define regional issues and support innovative initiatives.

Recognizing the Importance of and Providing Access to Nanoscience-specific Advice and Expertise

In 2004, PCAST was designated as the National Nanotechnology Advisory Panel[31] in response to the NRC report *Small Wonders, Endless Frontiers* and the 21st Century Nanotechnology Research and Development Act.[32,33] Although acknowledging designation of the nation's preeminent committee of science advisors to the government as a welcome testament to the NNI's importance to the country, the committee concluded that there is an ongoing national need for an independent panel of scientific and technical advisors with operational expertise specific to nanotechnology and nanoscience. Such an advisory panel would be available to provide advice to PCAST, the NSET Subcommittee, and the NNCO on research opportunities, investment strategies, approaches to responsible development, and program priorities focused on nanoscale science and engineering.

Specific activities of such a panel could include regular consultation with the leaders of federal agencies participating in the NNI to discuss and provide scientific and technical input and thus help ensure ongoing coordination of NNI program goals, budgets, and reporting. Such meetings could help to build additional new bridges among NNI-participating agencies and to proactively identify emerging societal implications of advances in nanoscale science, engineering, and technology—the committee has not seen any evidence of PCAST doing this.

The many advisory committees established across the federal government that operate under the Federal Advisory Committee Act provide multiple successful models for emulation in establishing this nanoscale-focused advisory panel. The committee believes that the President's Information Technology Advisory Committee, as it operated before its responsibilities also were assumed by PCAST, is a good model for a future nanoscale advisory panel.

The committee recognizes that PCAST in its role as NNAP created a nanotechnology technical advisory group (TAG) of about 50 government and private sector nanotechnology scientists to assist PCAST in its execution of its NNAP-related tasks. However, the committee agrees with assessments it received from many quarters that the TAG is not an effective mechanism and that a more focused and proactive approach is required. The committee concluded that the size and scope of the NNI merit a smaller, more structured and effective, dedicated advisory panel.

The chartering of a specific NNI-level advisory mechanism would provide the government the opportunity to establish a panel of experts optimized for addressing nanoscale R&D and nanotechnology issues specific to NNI goals rather than relying on the advice of the multiplicity of agency advisory panels that are focused on the mission needs of those agencies. Such an advisory panel would be well positioned also to provide advice on (1) prioritizing the support for short- and long-term research, (2) balancing the allocation of resources for large-scale centers and the work of individual principal investigators, and (3) giving expert advice on the value of high-risk but high-reward research requiring interdisciplinary expertise. Therefore, the committee offers the following recommendation:

Recommendation. So that a source of independent expert advice on nanoscience and nanotechnology is readily available to the NSET Subcommittee, the NNCO, and PCAST, the committee recommends that the federal government establish an independent advisory panel with specific operational expertise in nanoscale science and engineering; management of research centers, facilities, and partnerships; and interdisciplinary collaboration to facilitate cutting-edge research on and effective and responsible development of nanotechnology.

SUMMARY OBSERVATION

The committee believes that the NNI is successfully establishing R&D programs with wider impact than could have been expected from separate agency funding without coordination. The NNI's management structure involves both top-down leadership and broad R&D community involvement that can be characterized as grassroots or bottom-up support. Collectively, the sum of the effort has translated so far into tangible, but difficult to quantify, results. For the continued success of the program, arguably the most important factors may be ongoing federal government support for and commitment to achievement of the NNI's goals, which to a large extent also reflect broad national goals. Stability and continuity of the program will lead to future gains. As a long-term investment by the nation, the NNI requires the application of foresight and vision, stability in goals, and continuity in funding support to ensure realization of the benefits whose development the initiative is meant to catalyze.

NOTES

1. Nanoscale Science, Engineering and Technology Subcommittee, Committee on Technology, National Science and Technology Council. 2005. The National Nanotechnology Initiative: Research and Development Leading to a Revolution in Technology and Industry. Supplement to the President's FY 2006 Budget Request. March.
2. Current NSET Subcommittee membership consists of officials from the Departments of Defense (DOD), Energy (DOE), Homeland Security (DHS), Justice (DOJ), Transportation (DOT), Agriculture (USDA), Commerce (DOC), State (DOS), Treasury (DOTreas), Education (ED), and Labor (DOL), and from the Environmental Protection Agency (EPA), National Institutes of Health (NIH), National Aeronautics and Space Administration (NASA), National Institute of Standards and Technology (NIST), National Science Foundation (NSF), U.S. Nuclear Regulatory Commission (U.S. NRC), National Institute of Occupational Safety and Health (NIOSH), Consumer Product Safety Commission (CPSC), Food and Drug Administra-

tion (FDA), Intelligence Technology Innovation Center (ITIC), International Trade Commission (ITC), U.S. Patent and Trademark Office (USPTO), Office of Management and Budget (OMB), and Office of Science and Technology Policy (OSTP).

3. Public Law 108-153, available at http://thomas.loc.gov/cgi-bin/query/D?c108:4:./temp/~c108jIZb59::, accessed July 2006.

4. Such a panel had been called for in a 2002 NRC review of the NNI. In 2001, following a request from the White House National Economic Council and the NNI-participating agencies, the National Research Council (NRC) conducted a review of the NNI and an evaluation of the NNI research portfolio, the suitability of federal investments, and interagency coordination efforts. The resultant report, *Small Wonders, Endless Frontiers: A Review of the National Nanotechnology Initiative* (National Academy Press, Washington, D.C., 2002), was released in 2002 with 10 recommendations on the NNI. The NSET Subcommittee subsequently provided responses to each of these recommendations, which pointed to significant progress in recommended program areas (such as the interface between biosciences and support for instrumentation) and the steady development of an interdisciplinary research community, responsive to the needs of society.

5. President's Council of Advisors on Science and Technology. 2005. The National Nanotechnology Initiative at Five Years: Assessment and Recommendations of the National Nanotechnology Advisory Panel. May. Available at http://www.nano.gov/FINAL_PCAST_NANO_REPORT.pdf, accessed July 2006.

6. Nanoscale Science, Engineering and Technology Subcommittee, Committee on Technology, National Science and Technology Council. 2005. The National Nanotechnology Initiative: Research and Development Leading to a Revolution in Technology and Industry. Supplement to the President's FY 2006 Budget Request. March.

7. For more information on the program component areas, see in this chapter the subsection titled "Development of an Updated Strategic Plan."

8. K. Koizumi, Congressional Action on R&D in the FY 2006 Budget, American Association for the Advancement of Science, available at http://www.aaas.org/spp/rd/ca06.pdf, accessed March 2006.

9. See http://www.whitehouse.gov/news/releases/2006/01/20060131-5.html, accessed March 2006.

10. The workshop agenda and a list of participants are given in Appendix C.

11. Nanoscale Science, Engineering and Technology Subcommittee, Committee on Technology, National Science and Technology Council (NSTC). 2004. The National Nanotechnology Initiative Strategic Plan. Washington, D.C.: NSTC. December.

12. The societal dimensions component encompasses three subtopics: (a) research directed at environmental, health, and safety impacts of nanotechnology development and risk assessment of such impacts; (b) education-related activities such as development of materials for schools, undergraduate programs, technical training, and public outreach; and, (c) research directed at identifying and quantifying the broad implications of nanotechnology for society, including social, economic, workforce, educational, ethical, and legal implications. (Nanoscale Science, Engineering and Technology Subcommittee, Committee on Technology, National Science and Technology Council. 2005. The National Nanotechnology Initiative: Research and Development Leading to a Revolution in Technology and Industry. Supplement to the President's FY 2006 Budget. March.)

13. Nanoscale Science, Engineering and Technology Subcommittee, Committee on Technology, National Science and Technology Council. 2005. The National Nanotechnology Initiative: Research and Development Leading to a Revolution in Technology and Industry. Supplement to the President's FY 2006 Budget Request. March.

14. Nanoscale Science, Engineering and Technology Subcommittee, Committee on Technology, National Science and Technology Council (NSTC). 2004. The National Nanotechnology Initiative Strategic Plan. Washington, D.C.: NSTC. December.

15. This information was communicated to the committee through agency presentations and discussions during the committee's workshops.

16. The Wassenaar Arrangement was established as a means to contribute to regional and international security and stability by promoting transparency and greater responsibility in transfers of conventional arms and dual-use goods and technologies, thus preventing destabilizing accumulations. Participating states seek, through their national policies, to ensure that transfers of these items do not contribute to the development or enhancement of military capabilities that undermine these goals and are not diverted to support such capabilities.

17. J. Solomon, Praxair, presentation to this committee, March 24, 2005.

18. See http://www.nano.gov/html/res/SRC_ExecutiveSummary1.pdf, accessed March 2006.

19. See http://nano.gov/, accessed March 2006.

20. Director, Defense Research and Engineering, Department of Defense (DOD), Defense Nanotechnology Research and Development Programs, 2005. Washington, D.C.: DOD. May 17.

21. Asia Nano Forum, 3rd International Workshop to Develop a Global Nanotechnology Network, May 26-27, 2005, Saarbrücken, Germany.

22. Nanoscale Science, Engineering and Technology Subcommittee, Committee on Technology, National Science and Technology Council. 2005. The National Nanotechnology Initiative: Research and Development Leading to a Revolution in Technology and Industry. Supplement to the President's FY2006 Budget Request. March.

23. See http://www.ncnr.nist.gov/whatwedo.html, accessed March 2006.

24. See http://www.nano.gov/html/society/ELSI.html, accessed March 2006.

25. National Assessment of Educational Progress Achievement Levels 1992-1998. Available at http://www.nagb.org/pubs/sciencebook.pdf, accessed March 2006.

26. Highlights from the Trends in International Mathematics and Science Study (TIMSS) 2003, December 2004. Available at http://nces.ed.gov/pubs2005/2005005.pdf, accessed March 2006.

27. National Science Board. 2006. Science and Engineering Indicators 2006. Vol. 1, NSB 06-01; Vol. 2, NSB 06-01A. Arlington, Va.: National Science Foundation.

28. National Research Council. 2005. Rising Above the Gathering Storm: Energizing and Employing America for a Brighter Economic Future (prepublication copy). Washington D.C.: The National Academies Press.

29. See http://www.nsf.gov/discoveries/index.jsp?prio_area=10, accessed March 2006.

30. See http://www.nsf.gov/news/overviews/nano/index.jsp, accessed March 2006.

31. Executive Order 13349 was signed on July 23, 2004, to designate PCAST to serve as the NNAP.

32. National Research Council. 2002. Small Wonders, Endless Frontiers: A Review of the National Nanotechnology Initiative. Washington, D.C.: National Academy Press.

33. Public Law 108-153, 21st Century Nanotechnology Research and Development Act, January 2003.

2

Tracking and Benchmarking Progress

Nanotechnology is an enabling technology for advanced materials and products, and the U.S. national investment in NNI-related R&D (see Chapter 1 for more detail), coupled with U.S. industrial strength and economic infrastructure, promises significant returns for the United States. Other countries with excellent science and technology (S&T) infrastructure and well-coordinated nanotechnology initiatives are also expected to have similar or perhaps better programs in select fields. While speculative in places owing to the lack and generally poor quality of the data available for examination by the committee, the discussion in this chapter addresses the relative position of U.S. nanoscale R&D vis-à-vis that of the rest of the world.

Benchmarking of science and technology as applied to materials R&D[1,2] has shown that attempting to track data and provide a quantitative analysis in support of an objective international benchmarking assessment presents considerable challenges, and this is true for nanotechnology as well. In carrying out this element of its charge, the committee examined certain input factors and the output indicators that together illustrate overall trends. The inputs, or investments, made by a country include public and private funding, infrastructure such as facilities and instrumentation, and R&D focus. The outputs, or accomplishments, derived from the inputs include scientific publications, patents, other intellectual property and intellectual assets, new business formation, standards, trained researchers and an educated workforce, and national coordination to address, for example, societal issues.

PUBLIC AND PRIVATE INVESTMENTS IN NANOTECHNOLOGY

Funding

Investment in nanotechnology, including both public and private funding, is a major factor used to benchmark the standing of countries' support for nanotechnology R&D. According to Lux Research[3,4] and the President's Council of Advisors on Science and Technology (PCAST),[5] the United States is a global leader among governments funding nanotechnology (Figure 2-1). Nevertheless, it is difficult to compare U.S. public spending on nanotechnology R&D with funding with that of other governments because of differences in calculating and budgeting expenditures. For example, how various governments define nanotechnology, invest through combinations of public and private funding, calculate indirect costs, and report R&D cost factors, including researchers' salaries, can differ from U.S. practice in connection with the NNI.

Despite its current strength, the U.S. position in nanotechnology investment is being challenged as nanotechnology funding in other countries increases to similar levels.[6] Boosts in R&D budgets to $1 billion a year for nanotechnologies and materials in the European Union have been announced recently, and launches

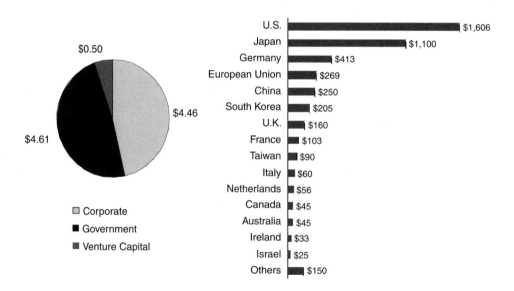

FIGURE 2-1 World nanotechnology funding, 2005. (Left) Nanotechnology funding globally by source, 2005 (U.S. $ billion). (Right) Government nanotechnology funding by country, 2005 (U.S. $ million). SOURCE: Lux Research, Inc. 2006. The Nanotech Report. 4th Edition. New York: Lux Research, Inc.

of new initiatives have been reported from various individual countries.[7] PCAST has commissioned the Science and Technology Policy Institute, a federally funded research and development center, to conduct a study to assess U.S. government funding as it compares to that of foreign governments.[8]

So that the current status of U.S. public investment in nanotechnology R&D can be better assessed, the committee in Chapter 1 recommends that the government continue to develop and improve means for tracking of agency budgetary requests, authorizations, and expenditures on an annual basis.

According to Cientifica's 2003 *Nanotechnology Opportunity Report,* global venture capital investment in nanotechnology-related companies totaled $261.7 million in 2002, with $207 million going to U.S. companies, $30.1 million to U.K. companies, $12.6 million to German companies, and $6 million to Israeli companies.[9] North America had the most venture capital funding up to 2001 (Figure 2-2), indicating that the venture capital industry is significantly more developed in the United States and suggesting the potential for ongoing U.S. leadership in venture capital-funded start-ups over the next several years. The committee notes, however, Japan's launch in 2003 of the Nano-Business Creation Initiative for the purpose of creating new nanotechnology businesses in Japan and building up the founda-

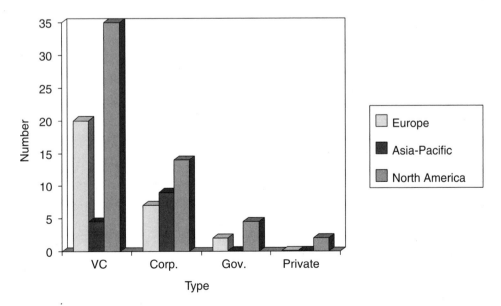

FIGURE 2-2 Number of venture capital funders by type and region up to the end of 2001. SOURCE: Cientifica Ltd. 2003. The Nanotechnology Opportunity Report. 2nd Edition. London: Cientfica Ltd.

tion necessary for its nanotechnology businesses to be global leaders in the future. Therefore, an increase in the number of venture capital companies in Japan investing in nanotechnology can be expected in the near future. Data were not available to it that would allow the committee to comment on possible directions in venture capital funding in other countries.

Infrastructure

In addition to funding type and amount, R&D infrastructure, human resources, industry infrastructure, and industry readiness also represent important investments in nanotechnology development. A recent survey by the Asia Nano Forum, presented at the Global Nanotechnology Network (GNN) workshop in May 2005, showed the United States as among the leaders in terms of funding for these infrastructure elements (Table 2-1).[10]

R&D Focus

Nanotechnology will provide a set of enabling tools, processes for manipulating matter, and new products and services based on nanoscale materials and processes, all of which will impact many industry sectors. Focused nanotechnology R&D funding by government agencies will enable improved positioning for business leaders and developers of platform technologies in government, academia, and industry.

Whereas the United States and the European Union as a whole are pursuing a broad spectrum of nanotechnology and related business areas, including nanomaterials, manufacturing, devices, energy, the environment, biotechnology/medicine, and instrumentation development, Asian countries have a more focused approach. According to an Asia Nano Forum survey, Japan, Korea, and Taiwan show significant interest in nanotechnology's impact on energy, the environment, and health care, and Australia, too, has a strong interest in nanotechnology in relation to health care (Table 2-2).

A 2005 report by the Asian Technology Information Program indicated that Japan had focused on research in nanomaterials, nanodevices, nanobiotechnology, and nanostructure characterization; China and India were more focused on nanomaterials; Korea and Taiwan had increased funding for nanodevices, nanomaterials, and nano-characterization; and Singapore had focused on nanobiotechnology and nano-characterization (Table 2-3).[11] It is noteworthy that Asian governments have supported nanotechnology R&D initiatives but that industry impact in Asia has been minimal, with the exception of Japan and Korea (see Table 2-2). The assessment presented in Table 2-2 indicates that public awareness in Asian countries of

TABLE 2-1 Asia Pacific Region Funding and Infrastructure Assessment of Nanotechnology R&D Compared with U.S. and EU Funding and Infrastructure

Country/ Region	Population (million)	Funding 2004 (U.S $ million)	Funding Per Capita	R&D Infrastructure	Human Resource	Industry Infrastructure	Industry Readiness
Australia	19.2	30	1.563	Good	Good	Fair	Fair
China	1282.2	60	0.047	Good	Good	Fair	Fair
Hong Kong	6.98	10	1.433	Good	Good	Good	Fair
India	109.5	5	0.005	In progress	Training	Fair	Fair
Indonesia	219.3	20	0.091	In progress	Good	Fair	Fair
Korea (South)	49.9	208	4.168	Excellent	Good	Good	Good
Malaysia	26.5	4	0.151	In progress	Training	Fair	Fair
New Zealand	4	11	2.750	Good	Good	Fair	Fair
Singapore	3.55	9	2.535	Good	Good	Good	Fair
Taiwan	22.8	91.1	3.996	Good	Good	Good	Good
Thailand	65.7	5	0.076	In progress	Training	Fair	Fair
Vietnam	82.85	1	0.012	In progress	Training	Fair	Fair
Japan	128.1	940	7.338	Excellent	Good	Excellent	Excellent
USA	296.2	961	3.244	Excellent	Excellent	Excellent	Excellent
EU	460	1,816	3.948	Excellent	Excellent	Excellent	Excellent

SOURCE: K. Tanaka and L. Liu, "Nanotechnology in the Asia Pacific Region," presentation to the 3rd International Workshop to Develop a Global Nanotechnology Network, May 26-27, 2005, Saarbrücken, Germany. Available at http://129.105.220.55/saarbrucken/saar_talks/Tanaka.pdf, accessed August 2005.

TABLE 2-2 Asia Pacific Region Assessment of Nanotechnology and Society Factors

Economy	Government Policy Awareness	Government Policy Support	Industry Impact	Education Program	Public Awareness of Benefits	Public Concern About Risk	Awareness of Energy Impact	Awareness of Environmental Impact	Awareness of Health Care
Australia	Medium	Medium	Medium	High	Medium	Medium	Medium	Medium	High
China	High	High	Low	Medium	Medium	Medium	Medium	Medium	Medium
Hong Kong	High	High	Medium	Low	Medium	Good	Medium	Medium	Medium
India	High	Medium	Low	Low	Medium	Fair	Medium	Medium	Medium
Indonesia	Low	Low	Low	Low	Medium	Fair	Medium	Medium	Medium
Japan	High	High	High	High	High	Medium	High	High	High
Korea	High	High	High	High	High	Medium	High	High	High
Malaysia	Medium	Medium	Low	Low	Medium	Fair	Fair	Medium	Medium
New Zealand	Medium	Medium	Low	Medium	Medium	Fair	Fair	Medium	Medium
Singapore	High	High	Medium	High	High	Good	Fair	Medium	High
Taiwan	High	High	Medium	High	High	Good	Good	High	High
Thailand	High	High	Low	Medium	High	Fair	Fair	Medium	Medium
Vietnam	High	High	Low	High	Medium	Fair	Fair	Medium	Medium

SOURCE: K. Tanaka and L. Liu, "Nanotechnology in the Asia Pacific Region," presentation to the 3rd International Workshop to Develop a Global Nanotechnology Network, May 26-27, 2005, Saarbrücken, Germany. Available at http://129.105.220.55/saarbrucken/saar_talks/Tanaka.pdf, accessed August 2005.

TABLE 2-3 Nanotechnology Funding and Projects in Asia

Assessment Criterion	Japan	China	Korea	Taiwan	Singapore	India
R&D infrastructure	10	5	8	7	6	3
Industry base	10	5	8	8	6	3
Manpower	9	9	7	6	4	7
Nano materials	9	8	7	6	5	5
Nano device	9	5	8	7	5	3
Nanobio	9	4	5	5	6	3
Nano characterization	9	5	7	6	6	4
Overall assessment	9	6	7	6	5	4

SOURCE: The Asian Technology Information Program (ATIP). 2005. ATIP05.026: Nanotechnology in Asia—Funding & Projects, p. 4. Tokyo: ATIP.

the potential benefits of nanotechnology is higher than public concern about risks, possibly indicating enhanced public trust, knowledge of science and technology, and proactive parallel efforts to establish guidelines and standards.

BENCHMARKING OUTPUT: INDICATORS OF OUTCOMES FROM INVESTMENT IN NANOTECHNOLOGY

Two indicators of output from nanotechnology investment that can be evaluated are trends in scientific papers published and in patents awarded. Yet benchmarking output is difficult both because nanotechnology is still in the early stages of discovery and development and because, as with government investments, the tracking of indicators is complicated by countries' differing definitions of what constitutes nanotechnology and by lack of uniformity and consistency in what information is reported.

Even within the United States, it is very difficult to gather data on publications and patents developed as a result of NNI investments, as no central agency is responsible for the collection and tracking of this type of data. In the following sections, the committee discusses some studies conducted by various organizations and individuals that assess and analyze publications and patents as indicators of national standing worldwide. While the trends suggested by each are similar, the raw numbers differ from study to study because of different methodologies, criteria (e.g., definition of nanotechnology), and sources used (e.g., United States Patent and Trademark Office data versus results of surveys of individual companies). Nevertheless, the committee found it possible to draw some conclusions as described below.

Scientific Publications

An analysis of the number of peer-reviewed scientific papers in the Web of Science database[12] that were published since 1990 and contained the keyword "nano*" showed the United States as a global leader in that indicator of output (Figure 2-3). This analysis also showed that, although the number of U.S. nanotechnology-related publications had grown each year, the U.S. lead was facing significant and increasing international competition: of the total number of "nano" papers published globally, the percentage originating from the United States declined from 40 percent in the early 1990s to less than 30 percent in 2004.[13] Global trends described in the benchmarking report by Lux Research also indicate increased nanotechnology publication output by other countries such as China, for example (Figure 2-4).[14] In the high-impact journals *Science, Nature,* and *Physical Review Letters,* the United States continued to lead, authoring 50 percent of the nanotechnology-related publications in 2006 (which represented between 6 and 7 percent of total articles published; Figure 2-5), even though the U.S. investment in nanotechnology was only 25 percent of the global total. Over the same time period, however, other countries' shares of such publications increased.

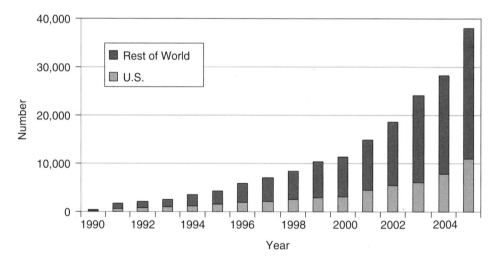

FIGURE 2-3 Number of nanotechnology-related publications by country of origin, 1990 to 2005. Number of articles in ISI Web of Science database found by searching on "nano*" as the keyword. SOURCE: Courtesy of James S. Murday, Naval Research Laboratory. Updated from a similar figure that appeared in President's Council of Advisors on Science and Technology, 2005, The National Nanotechnology Initiative at Five Years: Assessment and Recommendations of the National Nanotechnology Advisory Panel, May.

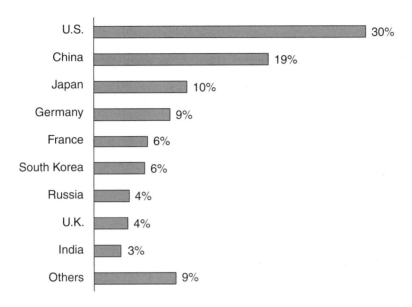

FIGURE 2-4 Percentage of nanotechnology-related publications by country of origin, 2005. SOURCE: Lux Research, Inc. 2005. Ranking the Nations: Nanotech's Shifting Global Leaders. New York: Lux Research, Inc.

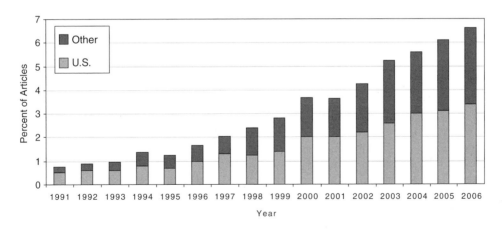

FIGURE 2-5 Articles identified by a keyword search on "nano*" as a percentage of the total articles published in *Science, Nature*, and *Physical Review Letters*, 1991 to 2006, and relative share of authorship, United States and other countries. SOURCE: Courtesy of James S. Murday, Naval Research Laboratory. Updated from a similar figure that appeared in President's Council of Advisors on Science and Technology, 2005, The National Nanotechnology Initiative at Five Years: Assessment and Recommendations of the National Nanotechnology Advisory Panel, May.

Patents

The number of patents applied for and granted is another indicator of a nation's standing and accomplishments with respect to R&D and business innovation. Yet, although patents relating to nanotechnology are currently tracked by the U.S. Patent and Trademark Office (USPTO), it is difficult to trace a patent back to a specific NNI-funded research project. Moreover, patents relating to nanotechnology might span more than one discipline or field, challenging the ability to classify patents and link them to particular research results. The use of a nanotechnology patent class created in 2004, USPTO Patent Class 977 (Box 2-1), has contributed recently to an improved capability to track nanotechnology-related patents in the United States.

Several analyses of data on patent activity have been conducted both in the United States and abroad. Huang et al. searched the USPTO database for patent titles and claims with nanotechnology-related keywords and found that more than 8,600 nanotechnology-related patents were issued in 2003 before Patent Class 977 was created. This number represented an increase of about 50 percent over the number issued in the previous 3 years.[15] The same study also indicated that the United States holds a strong leadership position with respect to patents in this area granted by the USPTO. In drawing conclusions about the U.S. share of nanotechnology patents it is of course important to take into account the concept of "home advantage"—that is, patent applicants are more likely to file for a patent in their home country rather than with a foreign patent office. According to Huang et al., aggregating the annual data from 1976 to 2003 showed that the top five countries receiving the highest number of nanotechnology-related patents issued by the USPTO were the United States (42,988), Japan (6,563), Germany (5,898), France (1,800), and Canada (1,772). In terms of share, U.S. entities accounted for about 67 percent of nanotechnology patents recorded in the USPTO over the same period. In 2003, the United States had 5,228 patents, followed by Japan (926), Germany (684), Canada (244), and France (183). Among the patents identified by that study's search, U.S. patents received the most citations in subsequently filed patent applications. Huang et al. also noted an increase in the number of nanotechnology-related patents issued by the USPTO to assignees in other countries, with the Netherlands and Korea showing particularly strong growth.

A survey by EmTech Research (a subsidiary of Small Times, Inc.) of U.S.-based companies, found that 25,372 patents were granted to 599 companies identified as nanotechnology suppliers.[16] Of these 25,372 patents, 2,063 (8 percent of the total) were for nanotechnology-related projects. The 599 nanotechnology suppliers (companies bringing products to market) were chosen by EmTech Research based on the following criteria: having headquarters or major business activity in the

BOX 2-1
USPTO Patent Class 977

In 2004, to improve the quality of its patent examination system in response to the rapidly growing number of patents relating to nanotechnology, the U.S. Patent and Trademark Office (USPTO) created a new U.S. Patent Classification Cross-Reference Art Collection (USPC XRAC), Class 977, focused on nanotechnology.

Currently, Class 977 contains 2,618 patents.[1,2] This class provides for disclosures[3] related to research and technology development at the atomic, molecular, or macromolecular levels, at a length scale of approximately 1 to 100 nanometers in at least one dimension, that provides a fundamental understanding of phenomena and materials at the nanoscale and enables the creation and use of structures, devices, and systems that have novel properties and functions because of their small and/or intermediate size.

In addition, disclosures in Class 977 may be defined by one or more of the following statements:

1. The novel and differentiating properties and functions of disclosures in this class are developed at a critical length scale of matter, typically less than 100 nanometers.
2. Nanotechnology research and development includes manipulation, processing, and fabrication under the control of the nanoscale structures and their integration into larger material components, systems, and architectures. Within these larger-scale assemblies, the control and construction of their structures and components remain at the nanometer scale.

In some particular cases, the critical length scale for novel properties and phenomena may be less than 1 nanometer or be slightly larger than 100 nanometers.

The novel properties or functions, e.g., special effects, are attributed to and are intrinsic at the nanoscale. Such nanoscale materials are infinitesimally minute arrangements of matter (i.e., nano-structural assemblages), have particularly shaped configurations formed during manufacture, and are distinct from both naturally occurring and chemically produced chemical or biological arrangements composed of similar matter.

Also encompassed within Class 977 are disclosures related to the controlled analysis, measurement, manufacture, or treatment of such nano-structural assemblages and their associated processes or apparatus specially adapted for performing at least one step in such processes.

Novel and differentiating properties and functions related to Class 977 must relate to the altering of basic chemical or physical properties of the materials involved as a result of their being assembled on the nanoscale.

---

[1]S. Maebius and S. Rutt. 2006. Simple steps make complex patenting system manageable. Small Times 6 (1; January/February).
[2]See http://patft.uspto.gov/netacgi/nph-Parser?Sect1=PTO2&Sect2=HITOFF&u=%2Fnetahtml%2Fsearch -adv.htm&r=0&p=1&f=S&l=50&Query=ccl%2F977%2F%24%0D%0A&d=ptxt, accessed March 2006.
[3]See http://www.uspto.gov/go/classification/uspc977/defs977.pdf, accessed March 2006.

United States; focusing on the development and sale of materials with features at a scale of 1 to 100 nanometers; developing these products as part of an integrated system; and demonstrating advantages inherent to these products or materials because of their small size.

A broader analysis performed in the United Kingdom[17] of nanotechnology-related patents awarded from 1990 to 2004 (Figure 2-6) used the keyword "nano" to select records without deleting those including words like "nanosecond" or "NaNO$_3$" that would likely reflect miscounts. The results indicated that the United States was the global leader in the number of nanotechnology-related patents held, followed by Japan, China, and Europe.

Cientifica's 2003 *Nanotechnology Opportunity Report* indicated steady growth globally in the number of patents relating to nanotechnology awarded between 1991 and 2001.[18] In particular, the years 2000 and 2001 saw surges in such growth. A 2003 review by Thomson Derwent of the number of patents in nanoscience and nanotechnology granted from 2000 to 2002 showed the United States as the leader internationally at 32 percent, with Japan, China, Germany, and Korea following at 21 percent, 12 percent, 11 percent, and 8 percent, respectively.[19]

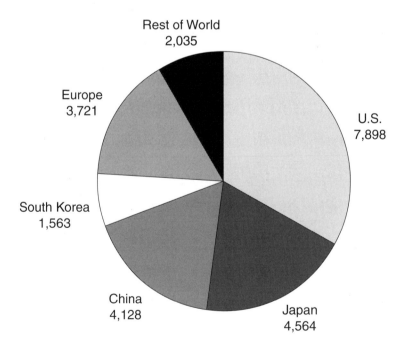

FIGURE 2-6 "Nano" patents awarded from 1990 to 2004 according to the applicant's country of origin.
SOURCE: Courtesy of N. Fox-Male, Eric Potter Clarkson LLP.

Drawing on USPTO Patent Class 977-related data in the Thomson Aureka and Delphion search engines and databases, a 2005 study from U.S.-based Intellectual Assets Inc. indicated that nanotechnology was a growing field worldwide over the period from January 1, 1975, to August 15, 2005, and also noted a significant increase in the early 2000s in U.S. patents issued; acquisition by U.S.-based companies of intellectual property (IP) in all areas of materials, manufacturing, and applications; and aggressive efforts by U.S.-based companies to follow up and block other companies' initial work.

At the 2003 GNN meeting,[20] it was reported that while the number of Chinese patents had increased significantly, the number of original inventions was very low. It was also noted at that meeting that very few Chinese patents were assigned to companies outside China.

In summary, a number of studies show that the United States leads the world in the number of patents awarded in nanotechnology, sometimes broadly defined. It is also clear, however, that U.S. dominance of the share of patents in this area is being challenged as activity generating intellectual property continues to increase across the globe.

Other Indicators of U.S. Standing

Other possible indicators of the relative position of U.S. nanotechnology R&D compared with that worldwide include trends in the employment and mobility of R&D personnel, attendance at international conferences, and data on the number of nanotechnology start-up companies. It is difficult at this time to benchmark with confidence the relative standing of countries based on such indicators, because trends usually become apparent only over longer periods of time. It might also be possible to gauge relative U.S. performance by looking at trends in the transfer of technology to industry. In this regard, a 2004 survey by the European Commission[21] indicated that North America was perceived as the leader in nanoscience R&D (67 percent) and in the transfer of nanotechnology to industry (66 percent) (Figure 2-7).

CONCLUSION

Input factors, such as investments and spending, and output indicators, such as publications and patents, can be tracked within the limits of certain constraints, as discussed above. However, linking these indicators to specific NNI investments is not possible with currently available data. In Chapter 1, the committee emphasizes the importance of consistent reporting of agencies' investments in nanotechnology R&D and recommends that the government continue to develop and enhance

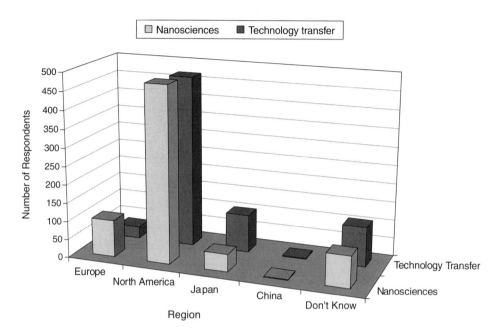

FIGURE 2-7 Regions perceived to be leading in nanoscience and the transfer of nanotechnology to industry, 2004. SOURCE: I. Malsch and M. Oud. 2004. Outcome of the Open Consultation on the European Strategy for Nanotechnology. Nanoforum.org. December. Available at http://www.nanoforum.org/dateien/temp/nanosurvey6.pdf, accessed August 2005.

mechanisms for uniform reporting and tracking of the funds requested, authorized, and expended annually. The committee believes that improved reporting of budget data will also help with tracing and elucidating the linkages between federal support for nanoscale R&D and output of the types discussed above to enable more solid benchmarking of U.S. standing globally. The committee suggests that an independent research organization could perhaps be commissioned under the auspices of the NNI to investigate appropriate techniques and methodologies for collecting and tracking data on output indicators that can be traced back to NNI investments.

Finally, the committee offers the following conclusion based on its analysis of the benchmarking data presented in this chapter.

Conclusion. *Although good comparative indicators of investment in nanotechnology R&D, resultant innovation, and economic exploitation of nanotechnology do not exist,* *existing data point to worldwide growth in investment in nanoscale research and innovation. The United States appears to remain in the lead, but with other countries closing this gap.*

NOTES

1. National Academy of Sciences, National Academy of Engineering, Institute of Medicine. 2000. Experiments in International Benchmarking of U.S. Research Fields. Washington, D.C.: National Academy Press.
2. National Research Council. 2005. Globalization of Materials R&D: Time for a National Strategy. Washington, D.C.: The National Academies Press.
3. Lux Research, Inc. 2006. The Nanotech Report. 4th Edition. New York: Lux Research, Inc.
4. Lux Research, Inc. 2005. Ranking the Nations: Nanotech's Shifting Global Leaders. New York: Lux Research, Inc.
5. President's Council of Advisors on Science and Technology. 2005. The National Nanotechnology Initiative at Five Years: Assessment and Recommendations of the National Nanotechnology Advisory Panel. Available at http://www.nano.gov/FINAL_PCAST_NANO_REPORT.pdf, accessed July 2006.
6. See, for example, Lux Research, Inc., 2005, Ranking the Nations: Nanotech's Shifting Global Leaders, New York, Lux Research, Inc.
7. S. Lawrence. 2005. Nanotech grows up. Technology Review. Available at http://www.technologyreview.com/articles/05/06/issue/datamine.asp?, accessed August 2005.
8. President's Council of Advisors on Science and Technology. 2005. The National Nanotechnology Initiative at Five Years: Assessment and Recommendations of the National Nanotechnology Advisory Panel. Available at http://www.nano.gov/FINAL_PCAST_NANO_REPORT.pdf, accessed July 2006.
9. Cientifica Ltd. 2003. The Nanotechnology Opportunity Report. 2nd Edition. London: Cientifica Ltd.
10. Asia Nanotechnology Forum, 3rd International Workshop to Develop a Global Nanotechnology Network, May 26-27, 2005, Saarbrücken, Germany.
11. The Asian Technology Information Program. 2005. Nanotechnology in Asia—Funding & Projects. ATIP05.026. Tokyo: ATIP.
12. The Web of Science database is maintained by the Institute for Scientific Information and contains data on papers in about 5,400 professional journals.
13. Note that the database search provides only the number of papers without indicating their relevance to the field, as might be indicated by a citation analysis, for instance.
14. Lux Research, Inc. 2005. Ranking the Nations: Nanotech's Shifting Global Leaders. New York: Lux Research, Inc.
15. Z. Huang, H. Chen, Z.-K. Chen, and M. Roco. 2004. International nanotechnology development in 2003: Country, institution, and technology field analysis based on USPTO patent database. Journal of Nanoparticle Research 6:325-354.
16. EmTech Research. 2005. 2005 Nanotechnology Industry Category Overview. Ann Arbor, Mich.: EmTech Research (a division of Small Times Media).
17. N. Fox-Male. 2004. Nanotechnology and patents—a European perspective. International Congress of Nanotechnology, San Francisco, November 7-12, 2004.
18. Cientifica Ltd. 2003. The Nanotechnology Opportunity Report. 2nd Edition. London: Cientifica Ltd.
19. Nanotechnology Research Institute. 2004. Asia Pacific Nanotech Weekly, Vol. 2, article 24. Available at http://www.nanoworld.jp/apnw/articles/library2/pdf/2-24.pdf, accessed August 2005.

20. International Union of Materials Research Societies. Undated. 2nd Workshop on Nanotechnology Networking and International Cooperation, October 11-12, 2003, Yokohama, Japan. Available at http://www.nims.go.jp/ws-nanonet/2_Report/NanoNetWS_RepLet0.pdf.

21. Outcome of the Open Consultation on the European Strategy for Nanotechnology. Nanoforum. org. December 2004. Available at http://www.nanoforum.org/dateien/temp/nanosurvey6.pdf, accessed August 2005.

3

Economic Impact

Over the past half century, much of the growth in the U.S. economy has been in high-technology, high-value industries, such as information technology and biotechnology, whose origins can be traced to innovation and discovery made possible by government-funded basic research. Recognizing the promise of research at the nanoscale as a driver of similarly revolutionary technology advances, the government mandate to fund basic research under the National Nanotechnology Initiative (NNI) involves an expectation for significant outcomes—that a federal investment in NNI-related R&D programs will lead to results that increase the U.S. capacity to effectively address national priorities, meet economic needs, and advance societal interests. In addition to improving our fundamental quality of life as a result of positive developments in nanotechnology-related medicine, energy production, national security, environmental protection, and education, the commercialization and adoption of new technologies resulting from nanoscale R&D are expected to yield a positive economic return in the form of benefits such as the creation of businesses, jobs, and trade. As the NNI grows in magnitude and complexity, it is imperative that the nation be able to evaluate its investments in nanotechnology and analyze how the return on those investments aligns with national goals, including those goals defined in the strategic plan for nanoscale S&T. To this end, the committee was asked to analyze the current impact of nanotechnology on the U.S. economy.

It is important to establish at the beginning of this discussion of economic impact that efforts to analyze R&D's economic impact in other areas have often been hindered by a lack of metrics and lack of a comprehensive empirical framework.[1] Assessing economic impact is also challenging because of the complexity of forces that drive economic growth and the inherent uncertainty surrounding outcomes observed at a particular point in time. Moreover, in general the timescales from research-based discovery to commercialization of technologies are long, often 20 years or more, and as an enabling technology, nanotechnology in particular is still in its infancy. The timescales over which the cumulative benefits of nanoscale R&D will become apparent will vary, depending on the nature of individual industries and products and the kinds of developmental research and testing required, such as clinical trials. Also, the investment needed for change and the availability of sustained investment for long-term gain will be determining factors. Although it is clear that nanotechnology will have an impact on many applications and industries, how to measure its economic impact is not now clear.

THE NANOTECHNOLOGY EFFECT

Lacking data on R&D outputs and how they contribute to the production of goods and services, and how such outputs affect comparative advantage, the committee found its ability sharply reduced to conduct a rigorous analysis of the current impact of nanotechnology on the U.S. economy. A few studies have attempted to assess the impact of nanotechnology on the economy by developing their own metrics. In discussing one such study here, the committee acknowledges that the foundation for such estimates is very modest and that other studies might generate other estimates.

According to a report by Lux Research, Inc., released in October 2004, the nanotechnology value chain cuts from nanomaterials to nanointermediates to nano-enabled products.[2] Nanomaterials are nanoscale structures in unprocessed form, such as nanoparticles and nanotubes. Nanointermediates are products with nanoscale features, such as coatings and memory and logic chips. Nano-enabled products at the end of the value chain are finished goods incorporating nanotechnology, such as cars and computers. In addition, the Lux report differentiated between "established" and "emerging" nanotechnologies. It defined established nanotechnologies as coming from well-understood processes, used for decades, which happen to yield products with nanoscale features. Examples include synthetic zeolites, high-strength metallic alloys, and microchips with feature sizes of less than 100 nanometers. Emerging nanotechnologies were defined as resulting from innovations using nanomaterials and nanointermediates, such as quantum dots, fullerenes, and nano-delivered drugs.

The 2004 Lux report estimated that nanotechnology accounted for $158 billion in global product revenue in 2004, with 92 percent ($146 billion) stemming from established materials and processes.[3] According to that report, only a small fraction—less than $13 billion—of 2004 product revenues came from sales of innovative, emerging nanotechnologies, with $12 billion of those sales deriving from nano-enabled products. The Lux report predicted that by 2014, emerging nanotechnologies would be incorporated into all computers and consumer electronics devices, 23 percent of drugs, and 21 percent of automobiles and that nanotechnologies would result in $2.6 trillion in product revenue corresponding to 15 percent of global gross manufacturing output. It also predicted that products incorporating emerging nanotechnologies would constitute $920 billion in value added, accounting for 2 percent of global gross domestic product. The committee could not verify the basis for these estimates or determine how they might compare with other figures.

The 2004 Lux report estimated that the number of new jobs created by nanotechnology was relatively small in 2004, with approximately 1,200 nanotechnology start-up companies creating about 6,250 positions worldwide, mostly for Ph.D. researchers, and more established corporations adding 3,000 similarly qualified workers worldwide. Although the number of R&D jobs increased slightly in 2004, the number of manufacturing jobs did not change, suggesting that workers already employed in manufacturing jobs were transferred to jobs involving the manufacture of nano-enabled products. The Lux report did forecast that the number of manufacturing jobs involving nano-enabled products would grow in the next 10 years.

The committee notes, however, that nanotechnology, like virtually all other disruptive or enabling technologies, will lead to the destruction as well as the creation of jobs. The Lux report noted that as emerging nanotechnologies develop and come to market, improved nanotechnology products will also drive second- and third-order disruptions across industries. The resulting impacts will be challenging to predict. For instance, the availability of new nano-enabled lubricants that reduce maintenance requirements could lead to a significant decrease in the demand for auto services, but a decrease in demand for lower-value maintenance services could be offset by the benefits associated with production of lubricants Given that nanotechnology is now still in the earliest stages of discovery and development, assessing its economic impact is speculative, although the importance of developing measurable relevant indicators is clear.

An indication of the future trajectory of nanotechnology product development was provided to the committee by M.C. Roco of the National Science Foundation, who has described four overlapping generations of new nanotechnology products that can be expected to evolve from the systematic control and manufacture at the nanoscale.[4] The first generation of products began to appear in 2001 in the form of passive nanostructures such as nanostructured coatings composed of dispersed nanoparticles and bulk materials such as nanostructured metals, polymers, and ceramics. The second generation of products, which appeared starting in about 2005, includes active nanostructures such as transistors, amplifiers, targeted drugs and chemicals, actuators, and adaptive structures; the key focus of research for this generation of products is novel devices and device system architectures. A third generation of products, expected around 2010, will comprise three-dimensional nanosystems and systems of nanosystems capable of various synthesis and assembling techniques, for which the focus of research will be heterogeneous nanostructures and supramolecular systems engineering. A fourth generation of products anticipated around 2015 will be based on heterogeneous molecular nanosystems, each molecule of which will have a specific structure and role; the focus of research will be manipulation at the level of atoms for the design of molecules and supramolecular systems, as well as characterization of the dynamics of a single molecule and the design of molecular machines.

An analysis by Cientifica estimated that capacity utilization in the manufacture of one first-generation product—nanotubes—was at no more than 50 percent, perhaps as a result of high rates of investment and limited commercial demand at present.[5] It is thus likely that for capital invested in the production of nanotubes, the current returns are very low or negative. How should economic effects be calculated for production activities that are yielding negative or very low near-term profits? Approaches such as attempting to value the intellectual property being created as a result of R&D leading to currently available nanotechnology products might give a different perspective on the returns to be expected from early-stage nanotechnology investments.

TECHNOLOGY TRANSFER

Source and Nature of Current Data

Technology transfer is an essential step in realizing a positive economic benefit from technology development, and measuring the progress of transitioning technology into the private sector is possible. For example, from 1987 to 2002, under the mandate of the Stevenson-Wydler Technology Innovation Act of 1980, the Office of Technology Policy at the Department of Commerce prepared biennial reports on progress in the transfer of technology from federal laboratories. Under the Stevenson-Wydler Act as revised in 2000, the reporting process was changed, requiring each federal agency that "operates and directs federal laboratories . . . to provide the Office of Management and Budget with an annual report on its technology transfer plans and recent achievements as part of its annual budget submission."[6] As part of its reporting, each agency now provides statistics for a core set of technology transfer indicators, such as cooperative research and development agreements, invention disclosures, patent applications and awards, and licensing agreements. The Department of Commerce (DOC) then prepares an overall assessment for the President and Congress based on the information in these federal agency reports.

According to the DOC's December 2004 report, which brought together the data on technology transfer from the agencies and also responded to a May 2003 PCAST report,[7] federal technology transfer indicators for all science and technology for selected agencies in FY 2003 (Table 3-1) showed that the top five agencies for inventions disclosed, patent applications filed, and patents issued were the Department of Defense (DOD), Department of Energy (DOE), Department of Health and Human Services (HHS), National Aeronautics and Space Administration (NASA), and the U.S. Department of Agriculture (USDA). However, because these indicators of output are not tracked against funding inputs by the individual agencies—and notwithstanding the inherent difficulties in valuing technology transfer and its effects—it is not possible now to link the NNI-related funding from these various agencies to the data collected on indicators of technology transfer. A complete analysis of technology transfer and its effects on the economy requires a capability for making such linkages and would also benefit from an ability to link data on research funding with data on publications or patents, given that publishing papers allows for the distribution of knowledge developed under the NNI and that acquiring patents resulting from research funded under the NNI could protect the research results as a valuable asset for further exclusive use by selected licensees.

TABLE 3-1 Federal Technology Transfer Indicators for All Science and Technology for Selected Agencies, FY 2003

Federal Agency	Inventions Disclosed		Patent Applications		Patent Distribution	
	Number	Percent Distribution	Number	Percent Distribution	Number	Percent Distribution
All 10 reporting	4,438	100.0	2,242	100.0	1,607	100.0
Top 5	4,130	95.0	2,178	97.1	1,582	98.4
DOD	1,332	30.6	810	36.1	619	38.5
DOE	1,469	33.8	866	38.6	627	39.0
HHS	472	10.9	279	12.4	136	8.5
NASA	736	16.9	163	7.3	136	8.5
USDA	121	2.8	60	2.7	64	4.0

SOURCE: Office of the Secretary, U.S. Department of Commerce. 2004. Summary Report on Federal Laboratory Technology Transfer: FY 2003 Activity Metrics and Outcomes. 2004 Report to the President and the Congress Under the Technology Transfer and Commercialization Act. December.

Broader Efforts Toward Technology Transfer

From a broader perspective the committee notes that the federal government has played a role in assisting companies, in particular small start-ups, to cross the significant gap between technology development and product commercialization, the so called "valley of death." The Small Business Innovation Research (SBIR) and Small Business Technology Transfer (STTR) grants[8] reserved for small businesses are designed specifically to help bridge this gap while meeting the government's R&D needs. The new STTR program focuses on expansion of the public and private sector partnership to include joint venture opportunities for small business and nonprofit research institutions, including universities. Under the SBIR program, each participating agency with an annual extramural R&D budget of more than $100 million must allocate 2.5 percent of its R&D budget for SBIR funding. Under the STTR program, the participating agencies whose extramural R&D budgets total more than $1 billion must allocate 0.3 percent (doubled in FY 2004 from the previous allocation of 0.15 percent) to aid in collaborative efforts between small businesses and non-profit research institutions.

Many start-up companies conducting nanoscale R&D have utilized SBIR grants, and the funds have been described as "crucial" for developing an economically viable product or technology.[9] This type of early-stage development funding differs from the funding for commercialization that venture capital might provide, in that it allows a much longer time frame for a return on investment. Some commentators object to restrictions on SBIR funding that prevent access by companies that have received venture capital investment.[10]

Other government programs for bridging the "valley of death" have included the Advanced Technology Program,[11] which was administered by the National Institute of Standards and Technology (NIST) and was designed to help industry invest in longer-term and higher-risk research with the goal of accelerating the development of early-stage, innovative technologies. The major emphasis of the DOD's Advanced Concept Technology Demonstration program, which focuses on technology assessment and integration rather than technology development,[12] is to help expedite the transition of maturing technologies from developers to users by demonstrating the initial operational capability of research concepts prior to their transition to acquisition and fielding.

The committee believes that productive partnerships between industry and government will be an important component in the successful commercialization of nanotechnology.[13] While government may invest in a variety of R&D activities and technology transfer mechanisms,[14] it remains the role of industry to provide the primary support and funding for commercialization activities. Public–private partnerships, however, can leverage the resources at academic and federal laboratories and also mitigate risks and maximize the outputs from expenditures on basic research.[15] A positive atmosphere in which companies can work with the recipients of NNI research funding can produce a multiplier effect that will increase and nurture nanotechnology innovation.

Partnerships between federal and state-level entities are also part of this positive atmosphere. In addition to federal–state partnerships, industry–state partnerships are essential to launching nanotechnology initiatives at the state level, as indicated at the 2003 NNI Workshop on Regional and State Programs.[16] State investments in nanotechnology include state–corporate partnerships, state–university partnerships, and partnerships with consortiums of corporations. It is worth noting, however, that on occasion disputes over intellectual property ownership have been a barrier to the successful implementation of these kinds of partnerships.

An example of state activity is provided by New York. Albany NanoTech, one of the world's largest centers for nanotechnology R&D, houses the New York State Center of Excellence in Nanotechnology and Nanoscience, the New York State Center for Advanced Technology in Nanomaterials and Nanoelectronics, and the northeastern headquarters of International SEMATECH, the research arm of the Semiconductor Industry Association.[17] Albany NanoTech is based at the University of Albany-SUNY and supports accelerated commercialization of high-technology products. More than 100 companies have partnerships and collaborations with Albany Nanotech, which "helps companies overcome technical, market and business development barriers through technology incubation, pilot prototyping and test-bed integration support leading to targeted deployment of nanotechnology-based products."[18] To date, these industrial and research partnerships and collaborations have yielded $1.6 billion in investments toward developing facilities, tools, and knowledge at Albany Nanotech that provide small, medium, and large companies with R&D programs access to these resources to serve their near-term and long-term technology development needs. This is a unique model involving collaborations among state and federal government, academia, and industry.

The first wave of innovations from nanoscale materials and processes is appearing in the marketplace, as reported by companies both large and small. Technological advances, while incremental, are stimulating vibrant activity at business forums and conferences. However, "valley of death" challenges remain, as does the need for continued federal R&D assistance in overcoming these challenges. Considering what is now known regarding the long timescales over which significant measureable economic impacts accrue from major R&D innovations, a sustained investment over many years from industry and government in support of the transition of nanotechnology to the marketplace will be required both to realize major economic benefit and to stay internationally competitive.

FINDINGS, CONCLUSION, AND RECOMMENDATION

Measuring Economic Impact

Evaluating the economic impacts of investments in nanotechnology R&D in a rigorous fashion will require a set of metrics and an aggregation of high-quality, uniform data on technology transfer and commercialization. Measures of intellectual property acquired and collaborative R&D partnerships established can also be useful to help gauge technology transfer activities in nanotechnology. For example, the potential for a financial return from patents held provides an economic incentive to individuals and corporations to innovate at the nanoscale. As discussed in Chapter 2, patents relating to nanotechnology are increasing in number, indicating that research results are leading to innovation. Applications for patents represent an initial step toward commercialization of nanotechnology and can serve as an indicator of economic progress, although patents serve as only one element of the entire technology transfer process.

In lieu of patents and other means of protecting intellectual property, some companies possess trade secrets to protect their technologies and products, but trade secrets are by definition impossible to track. Data on publications in scientific journals (see Chapter 2) are typical indicators of technical progress, but not necessarily of economic progress. Similarly, data on the recruitment of graduate students in nanoscale-related fields can be tracked, but it is difficult to link their work in this field to economic growth. Also, since nanotechnology is interdisciplinary and not yet a recognized field with a corresponding degree at universities, accounting rigorously for the number of students in nanotechnology-relevant areas is a challenging task. Today some data on cooperative research and development agreements, invention disclosures, and licensing agreements are being collected at the federal level as indicators of technology transfer. These data are not, however, being tracked for nanotechnology under the NNI.

While the reporting by NNI-participating agencies on federal funding of nanoscale R&D is an important first-order data point for policy and benchmarking, it does not yield information about state funding or private investments. In particular, R&D expenditures by industry are important for commercialization and realization of a positive economic impact. Although collecting workforce data from nanotechnology-based small companies is easier than measuring the jobs in large corporations that result directly from advances in nanotechnology-enabled products, currently jobs in nanotechnology R&D and manufacturing are not clearly reported. Sales of nanotechnology-enabled products can be tracked and possibly linked to data on the products that nanotechnology products are replacing, but the collection of these data is not widespread. While the number of nanotechnology-enabled companies is tracked, it is subject to varying definitions of "nanotechnology-enabled."

It is clear to the committee from its search for relevant data and metrics that the current quantity, quality, and nature of data on and indicators for tracking the economic impact of nanotechnology are severely deficient: the current data for tracking and assessing impact are unreliable, inconsistent, or non-existent, and many questions remain unanswered. Currently, there also tends to be too much forecasting based on assumptions and guesswork, and not enough on hard data or any rigorous empirical economic framework. Clearly, evaluating the economic impact of nanotechnology will require careful consideration of exactly how to measure the full effects of an emerging and pervasive technology, as well as assessment of the feasibility of developing, collecting, and tracking the relevant data and metrics.

Conclusion. *Currently, it is too early to gauge the economic impact of nanotechnology, which is still in very early stages of discovery and development. Moreover, any future analysis of economic impact will be hindered unless data are collected and metrics developed that will facilitate a rigorous analysis of economic indicators such as jobs created or individuals employed as a result of nanotechnology development. As both an enabling and a disruptive technology, nanotechnology will have effects that extend beyond one specific industry or market sector and will also be pervasive in multiple applications, a circumstance that will present additional challenges to rigorous assessment of the technology's economic impact.*

While it will be important for each federal agency to devise a set of data and metrics pertinent to its particular mission, some consistency and uniformity in reporting across the agencies will be important if future economic analyses are to aggregate data across the government. The committee believes that the NNI's demonstrated coordination capabilities across the NSET-member agencies will be critical to the successful development of the most relevant metrics.

Nanoscale technologies enable S&T progress and innovation with the promise of broad-based economic impact. Indicators must reflect the breadth of nanotechnology to capture the full benefit. Successfully developing metrics of progress, success, and return on investment could provide policymakers with the means to more confidently design and assess economic forecasts of the effects of nanotechnology. Greater emphasis is now needed to establish the foundations to aid future analyses. Given that nanotechnology is in its infancy, the timely development of indicators will facilitate the development of a more complete database of trends as nanotechnologies mature in the marketplace.

The committee concluded that currently available data are insufficient to permit a quantitative analysis of the economic impact of nanotechnology. In addition, those public and private forecasts of the impact of nanotechnology that are available lack consistency. The committee believes that the feasibility of developing methodologies and perhaps new indicators will have to be studied if high-quality data are to be available for future assessments of economic impact that are more quantitative than qualitative in nature. The committee therefore thinks that the NSET Subcommittee co-chairs should make a priority of studying whether a foundation of data to aid policy and decision makers in future analyses can be established.

Recommendation. To establish a basis for assessing the NNI's economic impact over time, the committee recommends that, as an initial step, the NSET Subcommittee carry out or commission a study on the feasibility of developing metrics to quantify the return to the U.S. economy from the federal investment in nanotechnology R&D. The study should draw on the Department of Commerce's expertise in economic analysis and its existing ability to poll U.S. industry. Among the activities for which metrics should be developed and relevant data collected are technology transfer and commercial development of nanotechnology.

The committee suggests that the methodology for any evaluation of economic impact should be broad and generic and might include, for example, best-effort evaluations of innovations in existing and new companies that have led to new products and new industrial processes. While these commercialization efforts are still in their early stages, it is important to initiate now the development of indicators for these activities and, looking forward, to maintain databases on the relevant commercial activities over the life of the NNI. Among the most important indicators are these: trends in nanotechnology-related intellectual property and other research outputs such as publications; the training of scientists, engineers, and technicians in nanoscience and nanotechnology; and technology transfer trends. The committee concluded that better data on technology transfer from R&D into commercial application are needed to understand and ultimately support realization of the societal and economic benefits of nanotechnology.

Defining and Assessing Progress

In addition to a substantial economic impact, many other results of the national investment in nanotechnology R&D are predicted that promise long-term returns for the country. For example, investments in national infrastructure—university excellence, student education, and national laboratory user facilities—will all have lasting positive impacts on nanoscale R&D in the United States and on the continuing U.S. capacity for innovation and future economic growth. The ability of a national initiative to inspire researchers to greater achievements, and especially to inspire students with as-yet-unidentified potential to study in this field, is almost impossible to measure but is nevertheless of clear benefit to the nation.

The benefits for the nation are likely to be greater because of the interdisciplinary focus of nanoscience and engineering. Students are now being trained across traditional disciplinary boundaries, and projects in universities and research institutes are being structured similarly. Now more than ever, industry values cross-disciplinary skills and seeks to hire researchers who have the ability to solve fundamental problems, who possess multidisciplinary knowledge, and who have a variety of technical experiences.[19] Many of the most promising innovations are a result of the application of interdisciplinary research. In the end, encouraging researchers to explore the areas at the interfaces of traditional disciplines may be the greatest qualitative contribution of the NNI, while NNI coordination across agencies to help shape and realize national priorities is likely to catalyze technology development of lasting economic importance. Benefits may range from advances in transportation and energy to benefits in human and environmental health. No doubt we will also benefit in a number of ways from a greater understanding of the world around us. Nanoscience and nanotechnology are making significant contributions in these areas, yet these contributions are difficult to tie to specific and measurable indicators.

NOTES

1. See, for example, Chapter 5 of National Research Council, 2005, Globalization of Materials R&D, Washington D.C., The National Academies Press, available at http://www.nap.edu/catalog/11395.html#toc.
2. Lux Research, Inc. 2004. Sizing Nanotechnology's Value Chain. New York: Lux Research, Inc.
3. Lux Research, Inc. 2004. Sizing Nanotechnology's Value Chain. New York: Lux Research, Inc.
4. M.C. Roco. 2004. Nanoscale science and engineering: Unifying and transforming tools. AIChE Journal 50:890-897.
5. A. Dunn, Cientifica, presentation to this committee, June 27, 2005.
6. Office of the Secretary, U.S. Department of Commerce. 2004. Summary Report on Federal Laboratory Technology Transfer: FY 2003 Activity Metrics and Outcomes. 2004 Report to the President and the Congress Under the Technology Transfer and Commercialization Act. December.
7. Executive Office of the President, President's Council of Advisors on Science and Technology. 2003. Report on Technology Transfer of Federally-Funded R&D: Findings and Proposed Actions. May 15.
8. See http://www.sba.gov/sbir/indexsbir-sttr.html, accessed March 2006.
9. NRC committee and staff discussions with Larry Bock, Nanosys, August 24, 2005, and Magnus Gittins and Michael Helmus, Advance Nanotech, September 7, 2005.

10. A congressional hearing on June 28, 2005, "SBIR: What Is the Optimal Role of Venture Capital?," raised such issues at the national level.

11. National Research Council. 2001. The Advanced Technology Program: Assessing Outcomes. Washington, D.C.: National Academy Press.

12. See http://www.acq.osd.mil/actd/, accessed March 2006.

13. NRC committee and staff discussions with Michael Idelchik, GE, September 6, 2005; Paolo Gargini, Intel, September 28, 2005; Larry Bock, Nanosys, August 24, 2005.; Magnus Gittins and Michael Helmus, Advance Nanotech, September 7, 2005; Amit Kumar, CombiMatrix, September 21, 2005; and David Macdonald, Nanomix, September 26, 2005.

14. D.C. Mowery. 2001. Using cooperative research and development agreements as S&T indicators: What do we have and what would we like? Strategic Research Partnerships: Proceedings from an NSF Workshop. NSF 01-336. Arlington, Va.: National Science Foundation, Division of Science Resources Studies. Available at http://www.nsf.gov/statistics/nsf01336/p1s4.htm, accessed March 2006.

15. NRC committee and staff discussions with Paolo Gargini, Intel, September 28, 2005; Larry Bock, Nanosys, August 24, 2005.; Magnus Gittins and Michael Helmus, Advance Nanotech, September 7, 2005; Amit Kumar, CombiMatrix, September 21, 2005; and David Macdonald, Nanomix, September 26, 2005.

16. Nanoscale Science, Engineering and Technology Subcommittee, Committee on Technology, National Science and Technology Council (NSTC). 2005. Regional, State, and Local Initiatives in Nanotechnology. Washington, D.C.: NSTC.

17. See http://www.albanynanotech.org/Programs/sematech_north.cfm, accessed March 2006.

18. See http://www.albanynanotech.org/about/index.cfm, accessed March 2006.

19. NRC committee and staff discussions with Magnus Gittins and Michael Helmus, Advance Nanotech, September 7, 2005; Amit Kumar, CombiMatrix, September 21, 2005; Uma Chowdhry and Krishna Doraiswamy, DuPont, September 23, 2005; and David Macdonald, Nanomix, September 26, 2005.

4

Responsible Development of Nanotechnology

Although the concept of responsible development of technology is frequently mentioned in government reports, industry publications, and the popular press, it is seldom defined. In the committee's view, responsible development of nanotechnology can be characterized as the balancing of efforts to maximize the technology's positive contributions and minimize its negative consequences. Thus, responsible development involves an examination both of applications and of potential implications. It implies a commitment to develop and use technology to help meet the most pressing human and societal needs, while making every reasonable effort to anticipate and mitigate adverse implications or unintended consequences.

The societal dimensions program component area of the National Nanotechnology Initiative (NNI) is defined as encompassing three subtopics: (1) research to characterize environmental, health, and safety (EHS) impacts of the development of nanotechnology and assessment of associated risks; (2) education-related activities such as development of materials for schools, undergraduate programs, technical training, and public outreach; and (3) research directed at identifying and quantifying the broad implications of nanotechnology for society, including social, economic, workforce, educational, ethical, and legal implications.[1,2] The committee's analysis of responsible development focused on current EHS research. Its efforts included looking at EHS-related activities and studies relevant to nanotechnology and examining some of the recently published work on toxicological and environmental effects of nanoengineered materials. In addition, the committee took note of efforts to address concerns about worker health and safety, including regulatory and standards-setting activities, as well as the importance of communicating about and involving the public in discussions of ethical and social issues in the responsible development and use of nanotechnology.

ENVIRONMENTAL HEALTH AND SAFETY

Nanomaterials have unusual and useful properties. But their unique attributes make nanomaterials a double-edged sword: they can be tailored to yield special benefits but also can have unknown and possibly negative impacts, such as unexpected toxicological and environmental effects. The environmental, health, and safety implications of nanotechnology are of significant concern to and a topic of serious discussion by government agencies and commissions, nongovernmental organizations (NGOs), the research community, industry, insurers, the media, and the public. A host of meetings and published reports have addressed EHS issues relating to nanotechnology, some of which are discussed below. EHS research published to date has provided some data indicating the potential for risks to laboratory animals exposed to nanomaterials and has shown that much more work is needed to assess the potential risks involved. Since much of what is learned as a result of EHS research will have a direct impact on R&D and manufacturing personnel who are initially exposed to nanomaterials, occupational health and safety risks, specifically in a workplace setting, must be considered.

Recent EHS-Related Activities and Studies

The federal government has committed resources to address such societal dimensions of nanotechnology as responsible nanomanufacturing and human health and safety. In 2004, memos from the Office of Management and Budget (OMB) and the Office of Science and Technology Policy (OSTP) to federal agency heads reiterated this focus, noting that "agencies should support research on the various societal implications of the nascent technology" by placing "a high priority on research on human health and environmental issues . . . [and] cross-agency approaches."[3]

According to the March 2005 supplement to the President's FY 2006 Budget,[4] $38.5 million was planned under the NNI for investment toward EHS R&D for FY 2006. In its role as the National Nanotechnology Advisory Panel, the President's Council of Advisors on Science and Technology (PCAST) defined nanotechnology-related EHS R&D as "efforts whose primary purpose is to understand and address potential risks to health and to the environment posed by this technology. Potential risks encompass those resulting from human, animal, or environmental exposure to nanoproducts—here defined as engineered nanoscale materials, nanostructured materials, or nanotechnology-based devices, and their byproducts."[5]

An ongoing EHS R&D activity involves the use of the National Toxicology Program (NTP) by the National Institutes of Health (NIH) to investigate the potential toxicology of nanomaterials and to initiate inhalation exposure studies for engineered nanomaterials such as carbon nanotubes and quantum dots. Another effort, at the Environmental Protection Agency's (EPA's) Office of Research and Development (ORD), includes the Science to Achieve Results (STAR) program. On March 16, 2006, 14 grants totaling $5 million were awarded to universities through the STAR program, in partnership with NSF and NIOSH,[6] for the investigation of potential health and environmental effects of manufactured nanomaterials. In addition, to date, EPA has funded 65 research grants for more than $22 million to study applications of nanotechnology to protect the environment.[7] Examples of results from STAR programs include the development of low-cost, rapid, and simplified methods of removing toxic contaminants from surface water; development of more sensitive sensors for measuring pollutants; green manufacturing of nanomaterials; and development of more efficient, selective catalysts. Other projects in ORD laboratories include research on nanostructured photocatalysts as green alternatives for oxygenation of hydrocarbons; studies of nanomaterials for use as adsorbents, membranes, and catalysts to control air pollution and emissions; and research on the effects of ultrafine particulate matter that could help inform research on manufactured nanomaterials.[8]

In other federal agency efforts, the National Cancer Institute (NCI), in collaboration with the National Institute of Standards and Technology (NIST) and the U.S. Food and Drug Administration (FDA), established the Nanotechnology Characterization Laboratory in 2005 to perform preclinical efficacy and toxicity testing of nanoparticles. In addition, the FDA has a grants program in support of orphan products research and development, but it does not conduct research in support of particular product applications.[9] Currently, the FDA's National Center for Toxicological Research is collaborating with the NIH, National Institute of Environmental Health Sciences (NIEHS), and NTP in evaluating size dependence on translocation of quantum dots in vivo and the phototoxicity of nano-sized titanium dioxide and zinc oxide.[10,11]

In its May 2005 report, PCAST acknowledged that current knowledge and data to assess the actual risks posed by nanotechnology products are incomplete. Furthermore, PCAST said that since exposure to nanomaterials is most likely to occur during the manufacturing process, research on potential hazards associated with workplace exposure must be given the highest priority. Also in 2005, the Nanoscale Science, Engineering, and Technology (NSET) Subcommittee formed the Nanotechnology Environmental and Health Implications (NEHI) Working

Group, which now involves over half of the federal agencies participating in the NNI. (See Chapter 1 for a description of all NNI's working groups.) The FDA is co-chair of the NEHI Working Group to develop new test methods and procedures to identify and prioritize risk analysis research.[12]

The NEHI Working Group provides an infrastructure for coordination within and between agencies, focusing on EHS research and programs relating to nanotechnology. Specifically, the NEHI Working Group aims to:[13,14]

- Provide for exchange of information among agencies that support nanotechnology research and those responsible for regulation and guidelines related to nanoproducts (defined as indicated above), to enable better communication of information on EHS issues relating to nanotechnology;
- Facilitate the identification, prioritization, and implementation of research and other activities required for responsible research and development, utilization, and oversight of nanotechnology, including research methods for life cycle analysis, and support the development of tools and methods to identify and prioritize risk analysis research;
- Promote communication of information related to research on environmental and health implications of nanotechnology to other government agencies and non-government parties, and support the development of nanotechnology standards, including nomenclature and terminology, by consensus-based standards organizations; and
- Assist in the development of information and strategies for safe handling and use of nanoproducts by researchers, workers, and consumers.

In June 2005, the EPA held its first public meeting about a voluntary proposed pilot program that would allow companies to submit information on the nanomaterials they are producing, how much is being produced, and possible worker exposure. On November 17, 2005, the House Committee on Science held a hearing titled "Environmental and Safety Impacts of Nanotechnology: What Research Is Needed?" to examine current concerns about environmental and safety impacts of nanotechnology and to assess the status and adequacy of related research programs and plans. NGOs have also been increasingly involved in addressing EHS issues. For instance, in 2005 the U.S. NGO Environmental Defense released a paper calling for the federal government to invest $100 million per year (about 10 percent of the NNI budget) in research on the potential environmental and health risks of nanotechnology for a period of at least 7 years.[15] In August 2005, the International Council on Nanotechnology (ICON), based at Rice University and affiliated with the Center for Biological and Environmental Nanotechnology, launched a database compiling publications relating to nanotechnology-associated environmental and health risks.[16]

The Woodrow Wilson International Center for Scholars and the Pew Charitable Trusts launched the Project on Emerging Nanotechnologies and, in November 2005, unveiled a database compiling global government-funded research on EHS issues relating to nanotechnology.[17] A 2006 report by Davies of the Woodrow Wilson Center argues that better and more aggressive oversight and new resources are needed to manage the potentially adverse effects of nanotechnology and promote its continued development.[18] In addition, in early 2006 the center launched a publicly available, online, and searchable inventory of nanotechnology-based consumer products.[19]

In October 2005, the International Life Sciences Institute (ILSI) released "Principles for Characterizing the Potential Human Health Effects from Exposure to Nanomaterials: Elements of a Screening Strategy," a paper by top toxicological experts that gives researchers the elements of a framework for assessing potential health effects from exposure to engineered nanomaterials.[20] It is noteworthy that the paper presents only elements of a screening strategy rather than a detailed testing protocol because of the lack of research data currently available. The paper focuses specifically on the need for thorough characterization of the properties of nanomaterials used in screening studies in order to obtain meaningful and useful results.

An update of a June 2004 report by Nanoforum, a networking activity funded by the European Union's Fifth Framework Programme, concluded that information and data are insufficient to accurately assess the risks of nanotechnology.[21] It pointed out in addition that many unanswered questions revolve around both the definition of nanotechnology and the framework of toxicity studies, and it encouraged continuing toxicology research. Swiss Re, a global reinsurer in the field of risk and capital management, published *Nanotechnology: Small Matter, Many Unknowns*, a report that addresses the risks and implications of nanotechnology, including EHS effects.[22]

Nanoscience and Nanotechnologies: Opportunities and Uncertainties, a report released in 2004 by the Royal Society and Royal Academy of Engineering in the United Kingdom, identified a need for more research to assess the potential risks relating to nanotechnology and recommended that the UK government establish an interdisciplinary program for research on the toxicological effects of nanotechnology.[23] The UK government's initial response[24] acknowledged the need for more research but did not lay out any plans for accomplishing it. However, on December 2, 2005, the UK government published a report that addressed the current state of knowledge on the potential risks of nanoparticles and identified areas in need of more research.[25] In another effort the UK Royal Society and the Science Council of Japan published a report based on a workshop they organized on EHS issues relating to nanotechnology.[26]

In summary, various activities in the United States and abroad reflect steps taken toward addressing EHS issues, but it is clear to the committee that there is still much work to be done. Ultimately, the studies and reports noted above suggest that there is a need for continued risk assessment and the establishment of regulations as appropriate, but more importantly, they also point out that for now there is very little information and data on, or analysis of, EHS impacts related to nanotechnology.

The Current State of Published EHS Research

The activities and studies mentioned above highlight some of the EHS issues relating to nanotechnology, but the body of published research addressing the toxicological and environmental effects of engineered nanomaterials is still relatively small.[27] As was pointed out by a workshop participant, two attributes of engineered nanomaterials are particularly important in relation to EHS issues—nanomaterials can enter the body, and their nanostructure can lead to specific biological activity. Such materials can include nanoparticles in the environment that can be inhaled or absorbed through the skin—such as aerosols, powders, suspensions, and slurries—as well as materials in the workplace that degrade during grinding, cutting, machining, or other occupational use.[28] What follows are some of the committee's observations on aspects of nanotechnology-related EHS research currently being reported.

A search in PubMed of the literature up to 2005 showed publications on the toxicological effects of two classes of particles—that is, chemically defined ultrafine particles (incidental, or naturally occurring) such as carbon black and silica, and intentionally engineered nanomaterials such as fullerenes and carbon nanotubes. The number of publications relating to incidental ultrafine particles exceeds the number relating to engineered nanomaterials by about 100 to 1.[29] Because of the discrepancy in the amount of toxicological data on each of the two types of particles and the unique differences in the particles' properties, data on incidental particles cannot easily be extrapolated and applied to engineered nanomaterials.[30] Now research to address the EHS impacts of engineered nanomaterials must thus be conducted.

In the small amount of research that has been done, there is evidence of adverse effects of engineered nanomaterials on laboratory animals.[31–33] For example, in two separate, high-impact studies, Lam et al.[34] and Warheit et al.[35] investigated the pulmonary toxicity effects of single-wall carbon nanotubes (SWNTs), intratracheally instilled, on mice and rats. Each concluded independently that these engineered nanomaterials showed unique toxic properties different from those of incidental particles such as carbon black, suggesting that it was the toxicity of these engineered nanomaterials, and not just the size, that presented potential EHS risks. In the study conducted by Lam et al., three different carbon nanotubes were used: raw nanotubes, purified HiPco™ nanotubes, both provided by the Center for Nanoscale Science and Technology of Rice University, and CarboLex, Inc.'s nickel-containing electric-arc nanotubes. In the work of Warheit et al., SWNT soot was generated via a laser ablation process and obtained from DuPont Central Research.

According to Warheit, health risk is a product of immediate hazards presented by, as well as the effects of longer-term exposure to, nanomaterials, and many different variables are involved in assessing toxicological effects.[36] For example, variables such as surface coatings of particles can yield different results from study to study, particularly with respect to toxicological effects.[37] Other variables that can affect toxicity include the surface charge and surface area of particles, differences in pulmonary response from species to species, the potential for particle aggregation and disaggregation, and whether the particles are fumed or precipitated. In particular, the absorption, distribution, metabolism, and excretion characteristics and toxicity of quantum dots have been shown to be highly dependent on both inherent physicochemical properties and environmental conditions.[38]

Developing a better understanding of the toxicity of nanomaterials also involves evaluating the effects of routes of exposure (inhalation, oral, dermal), the dose and magnitude of exposure, and the extent of biological response (local versus systemic).[39] For example, Semmler et al. and Elder et al.[40,41] found systemic effects that spread beyond the lungs of rats exposed to ultrafine particles by inhalation. In FY 2005, in collaboration with the EPA and NSF, NIOSH funded extramural research through a $7 million competitive grant to principal investigators conducting studies in the areas of fate and transport, and exposure to and toxicity of nanoparticles and nanotubes.[42]

In carrying out EHS R&D, it is critical to know exactly what is being characterized and to track apparent cause and effect relationships precisely and specifically Nanoscale particles and nanotechnologies differ and do not all fit under one giant umbrella with respect to predictions of their effects.[43] Classifying nanoscale particles and identifying relevant characteristics and properties are important steps in avoiding generalizations about all matter at the nanoscale. Information on the composition and structure of nanomaterials, purity levels, and well-defined controls and baselines must be known to identify potential risks.

An indication of the number of variables and degree of complexity involved is apparent in the above-mentioned study conducted by Lam et al. on the effects of inhaled SWNTs on mice: For example, the three types of carbon nanotubes used were each made by different methods and contained different types or amounts of residual metals. In addition, both negative and positive controls were used with the carbon black (Printex 90®), from Degussa Corporation, and the quartz (Min-U-Sil-5®), from US Silica, respectively.[44] Each of these materials has its own Material Safety Data Sheet outlining its specifications. The study by Warheit et al. cited above used SWNTs that were 1.4 nm in diameter and greater than 1 micron in length[45] and that existed not as individual units but as 30-nm-diameter agglomerates. The composition of the soot was 30 to 40 percent amorphous carbon, 5 percent each of nickel and cobalt, and the remainder SWNT agglomerates. Quartz particles in the form of crystalline silica (Min-U-Sil-5), from Pittsburgh Glass and Sand Corporation, and carbonyl iron particles, from GAF Corporation, were used as positive and negative controls, respectively.[46]

The number and types of variables in these two studies alone suggest the type and amount of work needed to ensure reproducibility of the results of these experiments, in particular, in regard to the nanomaterials used and the resulting specific EHS impact posited. That is, the experimental methodology should inspire confidence in the results, data, and conclusions.

The ability to carry out comprehensive EHS R&D requires that techniques and instrumentation for characterization and measurement be developed that will enable determination of the exact composition of a nanomaterial in a substance or product, as well as the physicochemical properties of specific nanomaterials. Chemical and physical data developed previously on chemically identical materials cannot be extrapolated to materials at the nanoscale, in part because bulk properties of materials significantly differ from the surface properties that are dominant at the nanoscale. Gathering relevant data specific to nanomaterials is essential to developing a relevant risk assessment process.

Most of the studies done to date have been conducted on laboratory rats, rabbits, and pigs, in which observed responses may differ from those in humans. Limited data are available on which to base predictions of real risks to humans; results of experimentation using animal models must be reproduced and extended in additional studies. Some preliminary studies have been performed in vivo in humans, including, for example, investigation of the effects of inhaled nanoparticles and ultrafine particles.[47]

In addition, work by Oberdörster et al., for example, suggests elements of a strategy for screening the toxicity of engineered nanomaterials that involves in vitro and in vivo assays of physicochemical characteristics.[48] In addition, the NCI Nanotechnology Characterization Laboratory also provides an assay cascade for characterizing nanoparticles' physical attributes, their in vitro biological properties, and their in vivo compatibility using animal models.[49]

Concerns for Worker Health and Safety

The laboratory or manufacturing environments are the settings where the initial contact between people—for example, researchers, technicians, and manufacturers—and nanomaterials occurs. Therefore, assessing risk as a basis for developing risk-management and risk-communication processes for the workplace is a critically important priority in the early stages of EHS R&D. As mentioned above, due to the potentially toxic properties of engineered nanomaterials, nanotechnology poses new challenges to conventional approaches to addressing occupational health and safety risk.

Proactive risk assessment and management of any technology require extensive strategic research[50] that could include such critical issues as assessing how toxicity differs as a function of type of nanomaterial, exposure route, dose, and biological effects and activity.[51] Understanding these issues requires the development of metrics for gauging exposure, methods and techniques for measurement and monitoring, and instrumentation.[52,53] In addition, the development of screening strategies and a framework involving elements such as those proposed in the work by Oberdörster et al. on toxicity screening for engineered nanomaterials can help in developing and evaluating the effectiveness of worker protection and workplace control strategies. Particular industries and working groups, such as the NNI-Chemical Industry CBAN group, could use such frameworks and help tailor them to specific sectors.

The National Institute for Occupational Safety and Health (NIOSH) has been providing national and world leadership in the responsible development and prevention of work-related illness and injury associated with nanotechnology.[54] In 2004, NIOSH established the NIOSH Nanotechnology Research Center (NTRC) to coordinate nanotechnology research across the institute. The NTRC's mission is "to provide national and world leadership for research into the application of nanoparticles and nanomaterials in occupational safety and health and the implications of nanoparticles and nanomaterials for work-related injury and illness."[55] Along with NTRC, which in FY 2005 funded five projects, other intramural nanotechnology research programs at NIOSH include the Nanotechnology Safety and Health Research Program under the National Occupational Research Agenda (NORA), which funded six projects, and the small NORA program, which funded one project. Under NORA, research has focused on characterization of the physical and chemical properties of nanoaerosols, their effects on health, and whether they present work-related health risks. In addition, other NIOSH divisions have funded intramural nanotechnology research relating to occupational safety and health.[56]

In 2005, NIOSH published a strategic plan for NIOSH nanotechnology research whose goals included preventing work-related injuries and illnesses caused by nanoparticles and nanomaterials; conducting research to prevent such injuries and illnesses caused by nanotechnology products; promoting healthy workplaces through intervention, recommendations, and capacity building; and enhancing global workplace safety through national and international collaborations.[57] To further encourage research on effects of nanotechnology on occupational safety and health, NIOSH published "Approaches to Safe Nanotechnology" to raise awareness of potential risks in handling nanomaterials and nanoparticles.[58] In that document, NIOSH requested data and information from stakeholders on the development of occupational safety and health guidelines and will be able to use that information to develop recommendations based on the best available science for working safely with nanomaterials. As new research developments occur, NIOSH will then update these recommendations and guidelines.

NIOSH has also established for public use and comment the Web-based Nanoparticle Information Library (NIL) (available at www2a.cdc.gov/niosh-nil/), which provides information on the physical and chemical characteristics of nano-materials, as well as their health and safety implications, to occupational health professionals, industrial users, worker groups, and researchers. The library contains images of nanoparticles, as well as information on the origin and synthesis of different kinds of nanoparticles, known applications and industries, and health and safety notes, including links to material safety data sheets.

Outside the United States, NIOSH and the UK Health and Safety Executive sponsored the First International Symposium on Nanotechnology and Occupational Health in October 2004.[59] The second international symposium was held in October 2005. In addition, NIOSH sponsored an international symposium, "Nano-Toxicology: Biomedical Aspects," in January 2006.

EHS Regulations and Nanotechnology

Notwithstanding the need for further EHS R&D as discussed above, there has been increasing initial consideration at U.S. agencies regarding regulation of the development of nanotechnology. In addition, the European Commission has also enacted new regulations. This section discusses some of these developments.

Environmental Protection Agency–Toxic Substances Control Act[60]

Under current TSCA guidelines, EPA must assess whether commercialization of nanomaterials might present a risk or potential risk to the environment and human health owing to the materials' unique physical dimensions and properties. A particularly daunting challenge is deciding whether a nanomaterial is a new chemical substance under the TSCA Chemicals Substance Inventory. TSCA defines a chemical substance as "any organic or inorganic substance of a particular molecular identity, including any combination of such substance occurring in whole or in part as a result of a chemical reaction or occurring in nature and any element or uncombined radical."[61] A new chemical substance is "any chemical substance which is not included in the chemicals substance list compiled and published under section 2607(b) of the TSCA Chemicals Substance Inventory."[62] Two nanomaterials that have the same chemical composition can have different chemical properties due to size differences, thus making it difficult to ascertain whether or not certain nanomaterials are new chemical substances. In addition, too little research has been conducted on environmental health and safety issues to assess whether certain nanomaterials are a risk or a potential risk to the environment or human health. Therefore it is not clear whether the TSCA in its existing form can address these challenges in nanotechnology.[63]

On June 23, 2005, in an attempt to address these issues, EPA conducted a public meeting on nanomaterials to discuss a proposed voluntary pilot program to collect information on nanomaterials that are manufactured, imported, processed, or used by companies.[64,65]

New European Union Chemicals Legislation—REACH

On October 29, 2003, the European Commission (EC) proposed a new EU regulatory framework for chemicals, COM (2003) 644. Under the new system called REACH (Registration, Evaluation and Authorisation of Chemicals), businesses that manufacture or import more than 1 ton of a chemical substance per year would be required to register it in a central database. The aims of the proposed regulations are to improve the protection of human health and the environment while maintaining the competitiveness and enhancing the innovative capability of the EU chemicals industry. REACH is designed to give greater responsibility to industry to manage the risks from chemicals and to provide safety information on the substances. This information would be passed down the chain of production.[66]

REACH shifts the burden of proof to industry to ascertain the risk of a material before it is introduced to the EU market.[67,68] The 2004 EC communication *Towards a European Strategy for Nanotechnology* called for risk assessment to be integrated into "every step of the life cycle of nanotechnology-based products."[69] In July 2005, the EC reinforced this idea in its action plan by stating that risk assessment should start at "the point of conception and including R&D, manufacturing, distribution, use and disposal or recycling" (Box 4-1). The action plan goes on to say that risk management procedures should be "elaborated before e.g. commencing with the mass production of engineered nanomaterials."[70] This statement suggests that

---

BOX 4-1
Life Cycle Assessment

Life cycle assessment (LCA) is the systematic analysis of the resources usages (e.g., energy, water, raw materials) and emissions over the complete supply chain from the cradle of primary resources to the grave of recycling or disposal.
—The Royal Society and Royal Academy of Engineering

Life cycle assessment is an important component of responsible development of nanotechnology; it requires paying careful attention to the full life-cycle risks presented by materials and products. Several nanotechnology-based applications and processes have claimed to bring environmental benefits, for example, through fewer resources required in manufacture or improved energy efficiency in use—or use of nanoparticles for cleaning up contaminated environments (soil, water).[1] It is important to make sure that there are net benefits over the life of the material or product and that issues of persistence and bioaccumulation are considered in such assessments.

LCA is now a standardized and accepted tool, covered by a set of international standards (ISO 14040–14044). The Royal Society recommends that "a series of life cycle assessments be undertaken for the applications and product groups arising from existing and expected developments in nanotechnologies, to ensure that savings in resource consumption during the use of the product are not offset by increased consumption during manufacture and disposal."[2] The Royal Society also notes that LCAs may produce results and trade-offs that have social and ethical dimensions.

---

[1]The Royal Society and the Royal Academy of Engineering. 2004. Nanoscience and Nanotechnologies: Opportunities and Uncertainties. London: The Royal Society.
[2]The Royal Society and the Royal Academy of Engineering, 2004; see note 1.

---

manufacturing and distribution of nanomaterials could be significantly delayed unless a company is able to demonstrate that a nanomaterial is safe.

At the time of this writing, the EC's REACH proposal is expected to be adopted by the end of 2006. Concerns have been expressed by EU member states, industry, and the U.S. government about the high regulatory costs and burdens that would be associated with the implementation of REACH, with estimates of €2.3 billion over an 11-year initial period and €50 billion over a 30-year period in direct costs to industry.[71]

U.S. Food and Drug Administration

The U.S. Food and Drug Administration (FDA) anticipates that many of the nanotechnology-enabled products that it would regulate will be "combination products," that is, drug-device, drug-biologic, device-biologic, or drug-device-biologic—products made of constituents that are physically or chemically combined, co-packaged in a kit, or separate cross-labeled products.[72,73] The Office of Combination Products was established in 2002 to develop policies and processes to clarify the regulation of combination products.[74,75] If a product meets the definition of a combination product, then that product will be assigned to a lead center within FDA. This assignment to a lead center would be based on the "primary mode of action" of the combination product. The May 7, 2004, *Federal Register* included a proposal for a rule that would define the primary mode of action as "the single mode of action of a combination product that provides the most important therapeutic action of the combination product."[76] In addition, the proposed rule described an algorithm that the FDA would follow to determine the center assignment.

The FDA regulates products only as a result of claims made by the product sponsor; that is, if a manufacturing company makes no claims with respect to a role for nanotechnology in the manufacture or performance of the product, the FDA may be unaware that nanotechnology is being used.[77,78] In addition, the FDA has only limited authority over potentially high-risk products, such as cosmetics.[79,80] Since little research has been done to assess the health risks of these products, many nanoproducts are not regulated. The FDA regards its existing pharmacotoxicity tests as adequate for evaluating most nanoproducts, but as new materials or new conformations of existing materials are developed that are identified as having the potential to pose new toxicological risks, new tests will be required.[81]

Consumer Product Safety Commission

Existing Consumer Product Safety Commission (CPSC) regulations and guidelines are being used to assess the potential safety and health risks of nanomaterials that are incorporated into consumer products. Under the Consumer Product Safety Act (CPSA), the CPSC can develop a standard to reduce or eliminate an unreasonable risk of injury associated with a consumer product.[82] Under the Federal Hazardous Substances Act (FHSA),[83] the CPSC can ban by regulation a hazardous substance if it deems the product to be so hazardous that the cautionary labeling is inadequate to protect the public. The FHSA defines as hazardous a substance that is "toxic, corrosive, flammable or combustible, an irritant, a strong sensitizer, or that generates pressure through decomposition, heat, or other means."[84] In addition, a substance may also be "hazardous" if the product "may cause substantial personal injury or substantial illness during or as a proximate result of any customary or reasonable foreseeable handling or use, including reasonable foreseeable ingestion by children."[85] Under both the CPSA and FHSA, pre-market registration or approval is not required, placing the burden of responsibility on manufacturers to ensure that their products are labeled as required by the FHSA.

In its 2006 Performance Budget Request to Congress, the CPSC identified nanotechnology as one of the emerging hazards in consumer products.[86] The CPSC has indicated that it will review and update existing chronic hazard guidelines to address the incorporation of nanomaterials and nanotechnology into consumer products. However, the assessment of health risks relating to nanotechnology is incomplete and inconclusive. Once these risks become well characterized and as proof of any hazards emerges, other regulations and guidelines, such as the Flammable Fabrics Act and the Poison Prevention Packaging Act, may also apply to consumer products in which nanotechnology is used.[87] The CPSC is also a participant in the NEHI Working Group to promote data sharing and best available practices for regulations of nanomaterials.

STANDARDS ACTIVITIES

In general, standards, guidelines, and best practices can create a framework for advancing the development of emerging technologies, while, at the same time, addressing and mitigating potential risks. As research in nanotechnologies progresses, information on health and safety and societal implications is being generated and examined, and potentially valuable data sets are being established. Government, industry, universities, and national laboratories all have a role in establishing standards for manufacturing, guidelines for safety and health, and protocols for the conduct of research—these are not the responsibility of any one single entity. Many of these stakeholders are engaging in the discussions and activities needed to provide the data, information, and ideas on which guidelines, standards, and practices can be based. These stakeholders include groups within professional organizations such as the American National Standards Institute (ANSI); government agencies such as NIST, NIOSH, NIEHS, NTP, and EPA; and a host of universities and industries, as well as NGOs and insurers.

The development of standards applicable to nanotechnology, including terminology and materials characterization and measurement, has been an increasing focus of professional groups in which activities have just begun. In 2004, ANSI formed the Nanotechnology Standards Panel (ANSI-NSP) composed of representatives from the national laboratories, federal agencies, academia, and industry. A draft charter was drawn up for the panel, whose mission was "to serve as the cross-sector coordinating body and provide the framework within which stakeholders can work cooperatively to promote, accelerate, and coordinate the timely development of useful voluntary consensus standards to meet identified needs related to nanotechnology, including: nomenclature and terminology, research, development, and commercialization."[88]

The Steering Committee of the ANSI-NSP has evaluated a proposal from the British Standards Institute (BSI) to the International Organization for Standardization (ISO) and recommended modifications based on public review comments. ANSI submitted its official position on the BSI proposal to ISO in April 2005. The recently created ANSI-accredited U.S. Technical Advisory Group to ISO TC 229 Nanotechnologies held its inaugural meeting at the National Institute of Standards and Technology in July 2005. More than 45 representatives from academia, government, industry, NGOs, and standards-developing organizations attended the plenary to formulate U.S. positions in preparation for the first ISO TC 229 meeting in November 2005 in the United Kingdom.[89] The American Society for Testing and Materials (ASTM) International has established the Committee E56 on Nanotechnology to create standards for nanotechnology. The committee encompasses over 100 organizations and individuals from 12 countries, including China, the United Kingdom, and Japan. The scope of the committee is twofold: to develop standards and guidance for nanotechnology and nanomaterials, and to coordinate with existing ASTM committees and standards related to nanotechnology. Subgroups have been formed to author documentation on terminology and nomenclature, metrology, and EHS issues.[90]

In anticipation of the impact that nanotechnology will have on the electronics industry, the Institute of Electrical and Electronics Engineers (IEEE) has partnered with other standards development organizations to develop certificates of compliance and standard operating procedures for high-volume manufacturing, to ensure reliable output, to protect workers, and to address environmental concerns. IEEE has developed consensus-based standards on how to electronically characterize carbon nanotubes. Because characterizing nanomaterials requires cross-disciplinary expertise, IEEE has worked with Semiconductor Materials and Equipment International and ASTM International to propose standards for the types and characteristics of nanoparticles, and nomenclature and terminology for nanotechnology.[91]

ETHICAL AND SOCIAL ISSUES

Although they were not a central issue for its deliberations, the committee recognized that addressing ethical and societal concerns pertaining to the emergence of nanotechnology will be an important part of responsible development. Currently, ethical considerations specific to nanotechnology have not come into focus, yet the concerns were articulated by experts in bioethics and engineering ethics and others[92–94] at the workshops held during this study (see Appendix D for examples). Although near-term and tangible ethical concerns related to use of nanotechnology have yet to be determined, it is not too early now to think about how to inform, communicate with, and engage the public to ensure broad consideration of what responsible development of nanotechnology might entail from a societal perspective.

One approach to addressing societal concerns involves application of the precautionary principle—the concept that action can be taken by responsible parties (such as government and industry) to prevent harm to human health or the environment even before certainty of harm has been established scientifically. At the 1975 Asilomar conference, for example, molecular biologists and geneticists developed a set of voluntary safety guidelines for the conduct of research on recombinant DNA[95] even as interest was growing in the potential for beneficial uses of recombinant DNA technology. The debate over and resultant approaches to addressing concerns about genetic modification of food items such as corn or soy are also worth examining[96–98] as efforts are made to integrate societal concerns into decision making about nanotechnology. A 2003 paper from the European Institute of Health and Medical Sciences, "Nanotechnology and Survival—Ethics and Organisational Accountability," suggests two components as important aspects of such efforts.[99] The first involves risk management based on an assessment of the novel behavior of nanomaterials in relation to human and environmental health and safety concerns,[100] and the second emphasizes accountability and giving the public a voice in making decisions about new technologies that will affect them and the fabric of their community.

In general, when the social impacts of a new technology are considered, ethics and fundamental research and development are treated as separate. Such an approach keeps facts and values separate, posits risks and benefits that are measurable and scalable, and assumes that uncertainty can be understood and managed scientifically.[101] But because nanotechnology is a potentially disruptive emerging technology, addressing its impacts on society will require a different approach. For example, to understand the structure, function, and effects of nanomaterials will require collaborations between chemists and toxicologists, as well as social scientists who desire to address the ethical and policy issues related to use of nanotechnology. Ensuring responsible development of nanotechnology will depend on taking an integrated approach to ethical issues that will also involve the public in thinking through the implications of nanotechnology.[102] Plato's observation that "the discoverer of an art is not the best judge of the good or harm which will accrue to those who practice it"[103] seems a succinct reminder of the value of informed outside review and societal participation in decision making about the introduction of significant new technologies into our environment.

Efforts to stimulate the public's participation can contribute to greater transparency in decision making and help forestall misinterpretation of information and subsequent confusion and fear of the unknown that can lead, in turn, to mistrust of both industry and government.[104] With the proper level of education, communication, and involvement, members of the public invited into the decision process take part as stakeholders in the outcome of future developments in a new technology. In the committee's view, public awareness and informed understanding of the risks and benefits of nanotechnology are thus extremely important, and they can be addressed in a variety of ways.

Among recent studies and activities pertinent to involvement of the public, the committee mentions two as illustrative:

- *Informed Public Perceptions of Nanotechnology and Trust in Government*,[105] from the Woodrow Wilson International Center for Scholars Project on Emerging Nanotechnologies, presents the results of a study conducted in May and June of 2005 of individuals' perceptions of government, nanotechnology, and regulation. Provided with information on nanotechnology and on U.S. regulatory and policy decision making relevant to nanotechnology, participating private citizens in Cleveland, Dallas, and Spokane, Washington, provided responses that included the following concerns:
  — Concern about the existence of hundreds of nanotechnology-enabled products in the marketplace and the expenditure of billions of dollars of taxpayer money on nanotech R&D about which people want to be kept informed and to have a role in decision making; while major benefits are anticipated, "government should not be making these decisions alone," especially with regard to medicine and food;
  — Concern about ensuring effective regulation, reflecting the feeling that voluntary safety standards applied to industry would not be sufficient to manage the potential risks associated with nanotechnology;
  — Concern that political pressure has interfered with protections for public safety and that regulatory agencies, although they were thought to be trying to ensure public safety, were being restrained by outside pressure from providing appropriate levels of protection; and
  — Concern based on industry's track record on past safety issues, arising in areas ranging from drugs to genetically engineered crops that industry has pushed products to market without adequate safety testing.
- In the United Kingdom, engagement of the public was sought via "Nanojury UK," an interesting approach in which 20 lay people received briefings on nanotechnology and after several months reported back with four recommendations for the UK government involving funding for the development

and availability of nano-enabled medicines; support for nanotechnologies that bring jobs to the UK by investment in education, training, and research; the need for scientists to learn to communicate better with the general public; and labeling for products containing manufactured nanoparticles to enable consumer awareness.[106]

Under the NNI multiple approaches have been sought to address ethical and societal aspects of the responsible development of nanotechnology, including education and public engagement. A study funded by the NSF and the Nanoscale Interdisciplinary Research Team (NIRT) at the University of South Carolina, entitled "From Laboratory to Society: Developing an Informed Approach to Nanoscale Science and Technology," focused on engaging the public in a dialog and providing educational resources to increase understanding of opportunities and risks involved with this new technology.[107] Two NSF-sponsored Centers for Nanotechnology in Society established recently under the NNI at the University of California, Santa Barbara and Arizona State University will provide a network of social scientists, economists, and nanotechnology researchers to address societal implications of nanotechnology.

Public perceptions are also influenced by the media's coverage of a technology. A report by Laing from Comex Research pointed to a general lack of coverage of nanotechnology by both Canadian and U.S. media,[108] and one by Friedman and Egolf of Lehigh University concluded that the number of newspaper articles about health and environmental risks was low in both the U.S. and British media,[109] suggesting yet another approach to improving knowledge and stimulating awareness and public participation.

CONCLUSIONS AND RECOMMENDATION

Based on its examination of currently reported research on environmental, health, and safety impacts of nanotechnology and the current status of regulation in this regard, the committee reached the following conclusions:

Conclusion. Notwithstanding the results of early research on the health and environmental risks of engineered nanomaterials, it is not possible yet to make a rigorous assessment of the level of risk posed by this class of materials. Further risk assessment protocols have to be developed, and more research is required to enable assessment of potential EHS risks from nanomaterials. The committee acknowledges that increased research on (1) health and environment implications and on (2) legal, societal, and ethical impacts will add to the cost of the development of nanotechnology. However, the committee concluded that the need for more EHS data requires an expanded research effort that will complement the important dialog on these issues that is being facilitated. At the same time, there is some evidence that engineered nanomaterials can have adverse effects on the health of laboratory animals. Reproducible and well-characterized EHS data will inform the development of rigorous risk-based guidelines and best practices, but until that information becomes available it is prudent to employ some precautionary measures to protect the health and safety of workers, the public, and the environment.

Conclusion. *Addressing the ethical and social impact of nanotechnology will require an integrated approach among scientists, engineers, social scientists, toxicologists, policymakers, and the public. Various studies have documented their participants' desire to learn more about the risks and benefits of nanotechnology and their willingness to participate in decision-making and regulatory processes to realize the full potential of nanotechnology.*

Assessment of the need for standards, guidelines, or strategies for ensuring the responsible development of nanotechnology is particularly challenging, given the unique characteristics and properties of nanoscale materials, the relative lack of data about potential risks posed by specific substances, and the convergence of nanotechnology with biotechnology, information technology, and cognitive science—each embodying its own set of compelling economic, societal, and ethical issues. The workshop discussions held during this study reflected the complexity of these issues. It was evident that participants saw in the development of nanotechnology a potential for addressing some of our most pressing societal problems—from treating cancer to meeting growing energy needs. At the same time, applications in health care and other areas present a clear potential for unintended and unexpected risks, as well as second-order consequences.[110] Some of these unexpected consequences may be beneficial, leading to innovations in currently unrelated fields. However, the possibility of unintended effects that may raise public concern demands proactive attention. Responsible development of these new converging technologies requires careful attention to social and ethical dimensions of their development and use. Sound guidelines and standards are imperative to minimize, for example, health and ecological risks.

There have been pockets of increased funding for EHS-related research. In the FY 2007 budget, President Bush proposed $8.6 million for nanotechnology research within EPA's Office of Research and Development, compared with the $4.6 million in the FY 2006 budget.[111] But although nanotechnology research benefited, there was a 4 percent cut in EPA's overall FY 2007 budget. As previously discussed, on March 16, 2006, 14 grants totaling $5 million were awarded to universities through EPA's Science to Achieve Results research program in partnership with NSF and

NIOSH.[112] These grants focus on the investigation of potential health and environmental effects of manufactured nanomaterials.

At the same time, a coalition of companies, NGOs, and the NanoBusiness Alliance trade group has called on Congress to increase funding for EHS research in nanotechnology. In FY 2006, 3.7 percent of the NNI budget was targeted for EHS research, with another 4 percent targeted toward research on ethical, legal, and social implications.[113]

It is also imperative that all stakeholders be involved in the risk assessment process. Given the rapid progress of nanotechnology, stewardship is essential in the form of addressing EHS issues, using nanotechnology for improving public health and environmental remediation, and managing nanotechnology-related risks. The responsibility lies with all stakeholders to make well-informed decisions that will lead to both realizing the benefits and mitigating the risks of nanotechnology.

In summary, the committee believes that EHS research needs to be accelerated and improved if the potential of nanotechnology is to be realized. In that regard, the committee offers the following recommendation:

Recommendation. To help ensure the responsible development of nanotechnology, the committee recommends that research on the environmental, health, and safety effects of nanotechnology be expanded. Assessing the effects of engineered nanomaterials on public health and the environment requires that the research conducted be well defined and reproducible and that effective methods be developed and applied to (1) estimate the exposure of humans, wildlife, and other ecological receptors to source material; (2) assess effects on human health and ecosystems of both occupational and environmental exposure; and (3) characterize, assess, and manage the risks associated with exposure.

The NNI's establishment of the NEHI Working Group has provided for exchange of information among agencies that support nanotechnology research and those responsible for regulation and guidelines related to nanoproducts. The NEHI Working Group also is helping to facilitate the identification, prioritization, and implementation of research and other activities required for responsible research on and development, utilization, and oversight of nanotechnology, including research methods to enable life cycle analysis. The working group has also served as a central focus for communication of information related to research on EHS implications of nanotechnology to other government agencies and non-government parties. The committee believes that such a government entity should continue to work with all stakeholders to proceed in an efficient and coordinated manner in addressing the responsible development of nanotechnology.

Finally, the committee emphasizes that EHS research that yields reproducible results and statistically reliable data will enable more informed discussions about how to (1) develop and disseminate EHS guidelines and best practices for R&D laboratories (including teaching institutions) and (2) regularly assess the adequacy and effectiveness of regulatory standards and policies for manufacturing facilities suc as industrial plants.

NOTES

1. Nanoscale Science, Engineering and Technology Subcommittee, Committee on Technology, National Science and Technology Council. 2005. The National Nanotechnology Initiative: Research and Development Leading to a Revolution in Technology and Industry. Supplement to the President's FY 2006 Budget Request. March.
2. The importance of addressing societal issues associated with the development of nanotechnology was discussed in the 2002 NRC report *Small Wonders,* which called for a "new funding strategy to ensure that societal issues become an integral and vital component of the NNI" (p. 3). See National Research Council. 2002. Small Wonders, Endless Frontiers: A Review of the National Nanotechnology Initiative. Washington, D.C.: National Academy Press.
3. Clayton Teague, National Nanotechnology Coordination Office, presentation to this committee, March 24, 2005.
4. Nanoscale Science, Engineering and Technology Subcommittee, Committee on Technology, National Science and Technology Council. 2005. The National Nanotechnology Initiative: Research and Development Leading to a Revolution in Technology and Industry. Supplement to the President's FY 2006 Budget Request. March.
5. President's Council of Advisors on Science and Technology. 2005. The National Nanotechnology Initiative at Five Years: Assessment and Recommendations of the National Nanotechnology Advisory Panel. May. Available at http://www.nano.gov/FINAL_PCAST_NANO_REPORT.pdf, accessed July 2006.
6. Environmental Protection Agency. 2006. $5 million awarded to study health and environmental effects of nanotechnology. Press release, March 16. Available at http://yosemite.epa.gov/opa/admpress.nsf/68b5f2d54f3eefd28525701500517fbf/6d536a255f4416848525713300520f80!OpenDocument, accessed March 2006.
7. Environmental Protection Agency. 2006. $5 million awarded to study health and environmental effects of nanotechnology. Press release, March 16. Available at http://yosemite.epa.gov/opa/admpress.nsf/68b5f2d54f3eefd28525701500517fbf/6d536a255f4416848525713300520f80!OpenDocument, accessed March 2006.
8. See http://www.epa.gov/ncer, accessed March 2006.
9. See http://www.fda.gov/nanotechnology/faqs.html, accessed March 2006.
10. See http://www.fda.gov/nanotechnology/faqs.html, accessed March 2006.
11. N.E. Alderson, FDA regulation of nanotechnology products, presentation at PCAST meeting, March 30, 2004.
12. N.E. Alderson, Nanotechnology Environmental and Health Implications (NEHI) Working Group, presentation to this committee, August 25, 2005.
13. See http://www.nano.gov/html/society/EHS.htm, accessed March 2006.
14. N.E. Alderson, FDA, presentation to this committee, August 25, 2005.
15. Denison, Richard A., Environmental Defense. 2005. A proposal to increase federal funding of nanotechnology risk research to at least $100 million annually. Available at http://www.environmentaldefense.org/documents/4442_100milquestionl.pdf.
16. See http://icon.rice.edu/research.cfm, accessed March 2006.

17. See http://www.nanotechproject.net/nanodb/, accessed March 2006.

18. J.C. Davies. 2006. Managing the Effects of Nanotechnology. Washington, D.C.: Woodrow Wilson International Center for Scholars Project on Emerging Nanotechnologies.

19. See http://www.nanotechproject.org/44/consumer-nanotechnology, accessed March 2006.

20. G. Oberdörster, A. Maynard, K. Donaldson, V. Castranova, J. Fitzpatrick, K. Ausman, J. Carter, B. Karn, W. Kreyling, D. Lai, S. Olin, N. Monteiro-Riviere, D. Warheit, and H. Yang. 2005. Principles for characterizing the potential human health effects from exposure to nanomaterials: Elements of a screening strategy. Particle and Fibre Toxicology 2:8.

21. Nanoforum. 2005. Fourth Nanoforum Report: Benefits, Risks, Ethical, Legal and Social Aspects of Nanotechnology. Second Edition. For more information, see http://www.nanoforum.org.

22. Swiss Re. 2004. Nanotechnology: Small Matter, Many Unknowns. Zurich, Switzerland: Swiss Reinsurance Company.

23. The Royal Society and the Royal Academy of Engineering. 2004. Nanoscience and Nanotechnologies: Opportunities and Uncertainties. London: The Royal Society.

24. HM Government. 2005. Response to the Royal Society and the Royal Academy of Engineering Report: "Nanoscience and Nanotechnologies: Opportunities and Uncertainties." London: HM Government.

25. HM Government. 2005. Characterising the Potential Risks Posed by Engineered Nanoparticles. London: HM Government.

26. The Royal Society and the Science Council of Japan. 2005. Report of a Joint Royal Society–Science Council of Japan Workshop on the Potential Health, Environmental and Societal Impacts of Nanotechnologies. London: The Royal Society.

27. A keyword search using "nanoparticles" yielded 101 global government-funded research projects currently in the Woodrow Wilson International Center for Scholars Project on Emerging Nanotechnologies database; 165 research articles in the International Council on Nanotechnology database; and 98 reports in the NIOSH Nanoparticle Information Library.

28. A.D. Maynard, NIOSH, presentation to this committee, March 24, 2005.

29. U.S. Environmental Protection Agency (EPA). 2005. Nanotechnology white paper (external review draft). Available at http://www.epa.gov/osa/pdfs/EPA_nanotechnology_white_paper_external_review_draft_12-02-2005.pdf.

30. V. Colvin, Rice University, Engineering safe nanoparticles, presentation to this committee, March 24, 2005.

31. C.-W. Lam, J.T. James, R. McCluskey, and R.L. Hunter. 2004. Pulmonary toxicity of single-wall carbon nanotubes in mice 7 and 90 days after intratracheal instillation. Toxicological Sciences 77:126-134.

32. D. Warheit, DuPont, Pulmonary impacts of exposures to nanoparticulates: Particle size and surface area may not be more important factors than surface characteristics, presentation to this committee, March 24, 2005.

33. U.S. Environmental Protection Agency (EPA). 2005. Nanotechnology white paper (external review draft). Available at http://www.epa.gov/osa/pdfs/EPA_nanotechnology_white_paper_external_review_draft_12-02-2005.pdf.

34. C.-W. Lam, J.T. James, R. McCluskey, and R.L. Hunter. 2004. Pulmonary toxicity of single-wall carbon nanotubes in mice 7 and 90 days after intratracheal instillation. Toxicological Sciences 77:126-134.

35. D.B. Warheit, B.R. Laurence, K.L. Reed, D.H. Roach, G.A.M. Reynolds, and T.R. Webb. 2004. Comparative pulmonary toxicity assessment of single-wall carbon nanotubes in rats. Toxicological Sciences 77:117-125.

36. D. Warheit, DuPont, Pulmonary impacts of exposures to nanoparticulates: Particle size and surface area may not be more important factors than surface characteristics, presentation to this committee, March 24, 2005.

37. S. Tinkle, NIEHS, Responsible development of nanotechnology: The toxicologist's perspective, presentation to this committee, March 24, 2005.

38. R. Hardman. 2006. A toxicologic review of quantum dots: Toxicity depends on physicochemical and environmental factors. Environmental Health Perspectives 114:165-172.
39. S. Tinkle, NIEHS, Responsible development of nanotechnology: The toxicologist's perspective, presentation to this committee, March 24, 2005.
40. M. Semmler, J. Seitz, F. Erbe, P. Mayer, J. Heyder, G. Oberdörster, and W. Kreyling. 2004. Long-term clearance kinetics of inhaled ultrafine insoluble iridium particles from the rat lung, including transient translocation into secondary organs. Inhalation Toxicology 16:453-459.
41. A. Elder, R. Gelein, M. Azadniv, M. Frampton, J. Finkelstein, and G. Oberdörster. 2004. Systemic effects of inhaled ultrafine particles in two compromised, aged rat strains. Inhalation Toxicology 16:461-471.
42. National Institute for Occupational Safety and Health (NIOSH). 2005. Strategic Plan for NIOSH Nanotechnology Research: Filling the Knowledge Gaps. Washington, D.C.: NIOSH.
43. V. Colvin, Rice University, Engineering safe nanoparticles, presentation to this committee, March 24, 2005.
44. C.-W. Lam, J.T. James, R. McCluskey, and R.L. Hunter. 2004. Pulmonary toxicity of single-wall carbon nanotubes in mice 7 and 90 days after intratracheal instillation. Toxicological Sciences 77:126-134.
45. D.B. Warheit, B.R. Laurence, K.L. Reed, D.H. Roach, G.A.M. Reynolds, and T.R. Webb. 2004. Comparative pulmonary toxicity assessment of single-wall carbon nanotubes in rats. Toxicological Sciences 77:117-125.
46. D.B. Warheit, B.R. Laurence, K.L. Reed, D.H. Roach, G.A.M. Reynolds, and T. R. Webb. 2004. Comparative pulmonary toxicity assessment of single-wall carbon nanotubes in rats. Toxicological Sciences 77:117-125.
47. Nanoforum. 2005. Fourth Nanoforum Report: Benefits, Risks, Ethical, Legal and Social Aspects of Nanotechnology. Second Edition. For more information, see http://www.nanoforum.org.
48. G. Oberdörster, A. Maynard, K. Donaldson, V. Castranova, J. Fitzpatrick, K. Ausman, J. Carter, B. Karn, W. Kreyling, D. Lai, S. Olin, N. Monteiro-Riviere, D. Warheit, and H. Yang. 2005. Principles for characterizing the potential human health effects from exposure to nanomaterials: Elements of a screening strategy. Particle and Fibre Toxicology 2:8.
49. See http://ncl.cancer.gov, accessed March 2006.
50. A.D. Maynard, NIOSH, presentation to this committee, March 24, 2005.
51. A. Nel, T. Xia, L. Mädler, and N. Li. 2006. Toxic potential of materials at the nanolevel. Science 311:622-627.
52. J. Solomon, Praxair, presentation to this committee, March 24, 2005.
53. C. Henry, American Chemistry Council, presentation to this committee, March 24, 2005.
54. NIOSH strategies for working with engineered nanomaterials can be found on its Web site (http://www.cdc.gov/niosh/topics/nanotech/), which has become a communications tool for public outreach.
55. National Institute for Occupational Safety and Health (NIOSH). 2005. Strategic Plan for NIOSH Nanotechnology Research: Filling the Knowledge Gaps. Washington, D.C.: NIOSH.
56. National Institute for Occupational Safety and Health (NIOSH). 2005. Strategic Plan for NIOSH Nanotechnology Research: Filling the Knowledge Gaps. Washington, D.C.: NIOSH.
57. National Institute for Occupational Safety and Health (NIOSH). 2005. Strategic Plan for NIOSH Nanotechnology Research: Filling the Knowledge Gaps. Washington, D.C.: NIOSH.
58. National Institute for Occupational Safety and Health (NIOSH). 2005. Approaches to Safe Nanotechnology: An Information Exchange with NIOSH. Washington, D.C.: NIOSH. October 1.
59. British Health and Safety Executive and U.S. National Institute for Occupational Safety and Health. Nanomaterials: A Risk to Health at Work? First International Symposium on Occupational Health Implications of Nanomaterials, Derbyshire, United Kingdom, October 12-14, 2004.

60. The Toxic Substances Control Act (TSCA) of 1976 "was enacted by Congress to give EPA the ability to track the 75,000 industrial chemicals currently produced or imported into the United States. EPA repeatedly screens these chemicals and can require reporting or testing of those that may pose an environmental or human-health hazard. EPA can ban the manufacture and import of those chemicals that pose an unreasonable risk. Also, EPA has mechanisms in place to track the thousands of new chemicals that industry develops each year with either unknown or dangerous characteristics. EPA then can control these chemicals as necessary to protect human health and the environment. TSCA supplements other Federal statutes, including the Clean Air Act and the Toxic Release Inventory under Emergency Planning and Community Right to Know Act (EPCRA)." See http://www.epa.gov/region5/defs/html/tsca.htm, accessed March 2006.

61. Toxic Substances Control Act (TSCA), 15 U.S.C. s/s 2602 (2)(a). 1976. Available at http://www.epa.gov/region5/defs/html/tsca.htm, accessed March 2006.

62. Toxic Substances Control Act (TSCA), 15 U.S.C. s/s 2602 (9). 1976. Available at http://www.epa.gov/region5/defs/html/tsca.htm, accessed March 2006.

63. A. Wardak and D. Rejeski. 2003. Nanotechnology & Regulation: A Case Study Using the Toxic Substance Control Act (TSCA). Washington, D.C.: Woodrow Wilson International Center for Scholars.

64. Environmental Protection Agency (EPA). 2005. Nanoscale materials: Notice of public meeting. Federal Register 70(89; May 10).

65. R.F. Service. 2005. EPA ponders voluntary nanotechnology regulations. Science 309:36.

66. European Commission (EC). 2003. The New EU Chemicals Legislation-REACH. Available at http://europa.eu.int/comm/enterprise/reach/index_en.htm.

67. M.C. Kalpin and M. Hoffer. 2005. Nanotechnology and the environment: Will emerging environmental regulations stifle the promise?" NSTI Nanotech 2005 Conference and Trade Show, Anaheim, Calif., May 8-12, 2005.

68. L. Koch and N.A. Ashford. 2006. Rethinking the role of information in chemicals policy: Implications for TSCA and REACH. Journal of Cleaner Production 14(1):31-46.

69. European Commission (EC). 2004. Towards a European strategy for nanotechnology. Communication from the Commission of European Communities.

70. European Commission (EC). 2005. Nanoscience and nanotechnologies: An action plan for Europe 2005-2009. Communication from the Commission to the Council, the European Parliament and the Economic and Social Committee, July 6, 2005.

71. M.C. Kalpin and M. Hoffer. 2005. Nanotechnology and the environment: Will emerging environmental regulations stifle the promise? NSTI Nanotech 2005 Conference and Trade Show, Anaheim, Calif., May 8-12, 2005.

72. See http://www.fda.gov/nanotechnology/faqs.html, accessed March 2006.

73. N. Sadrieh, FDA perspective on nanomaterial-containing products, presentation at Nanobusiness Conference, May 2005.

74. See http://www.fda.gov/nanotechnology/faqs.html, accessed March 2006.

75. N. Sadrieh, FDA perspective on nanomaterial-containing products, presentation at Nanobusiness Conference, May 2005.

76. Department of Health and Human Services, Food and Drug Administration. 2004. Definition of primary mode of action of a combination product. Federal Register 69(89; May 7).

77. See http://www.fda.gov/nanotechnology/regulation.html, accessed March 2006.

78. N.E. Alderson, FDA regulation of nanotechnology products, presentation at PCAST meeting, March 30, 2004.

79. See http://www.fda.gov/nanotechnology/regulation.html, accessed March 2006.

80. N.E. Alderson, FDA regulation of nanotechnology products, presentation at PCAST meeting, March 30, 2004.

81. N.E. Alderson, FDA regulation of nanotechnology products, presentation at PCAST meeting, March 30, 2004.

82. U.S. Consumer Product Safety Act (CPSA). Codified at 15 U.S.C. 2051-2084. Public Law 92-573; 86 Stat. 1207, Oct. 27, 1972.

83. Federal Hazardous Substances Act (FHSA). Codified at 15 U.S.C. 1261-1278. Public Law 86-613; 74 Stat. 372, July 12, 1960, as amended.

84. Federal Hazardous Substances Act (FHSA). Codified at 15 U.S.C. 1261-1278. Public Law 86-613; 74 Stat. 372, July 12, 1960, as amended.

85. Federal Hazardous Substances Act (FHSA). Codified at 15 U.S.C. 1261-1278. Public Law 86-613; 74 Stat. 372, July 12, 1960, as amended.

86. U.S. Consumer Product Safety Commission (CPSC). 2005. 2006 Performance Budget Request: Saving Lives and Keeping Families Safe. February.

87. J. Bromme. 2005. Nanotechnology and the consumer product safety commission. Product Safety & Liability Reporter 33(11; March 14).

88. F. Schrotter, American National Standards Institute, presentation to this committee, March 24, 2005.

89. See http://www.ansi.org/standards_activities/standards_boards_panels/nsp/overview.aspx?menuid=3#news, accessed March 2006.

90. P. Picariello, ASTM International, presentation to this committee, March 24, 2005.

91. D. Gamota, Motorola, presentation to this committee, March 24, 2005.

92. D.M. Berube, University of South Carolina, presentation to this committee, February 11, 2005.

93. D. Rejeski, Woodrow Wilson International Center for Scholars, presentation to this committee, February 11, 2005.

94. N. Jacobstein, Institute for Molecular Manufacturing, presentation to this committee, February 11, 2005.

95. D. Rolison, Naval Research Laboratory, presentation to this committee, March 25, 2005.

96. Rio Declaration on Environment and Development. 1992. The United Nations Conference on Environment and Development, Rio de Janeiro, Brazil.

97. National Research Council. 1989. Field Testing Genetically Modified Organisms: Framework for Decisions. Washington, D.C.: National Academy Press.

98. Institute of Medicine and National Research Council. 2004. Safety of Genetically Engineered Foods: Approaches to Assessing Unintended Health Effects. Washington, D.C.: The National Academies Press.

99. G. Hunt, Nanotechnology and survival—Ethics and organisational accountability, paper delivered at the Institute for Seizon and the Life Sciences, July 5, 2003, Tokyo. Available at http://www.freedomtocare.org/page316.htm.

100. In this regard, the committee notes that NNI-participating agencies are funding research on the novel properties and biological and environmental effects of some nanomaterials that have already been introduced into the environment.

101. G. Khushf, University of South Carolina, presentation to this committee, March 25, 2005.

102. G. Khushf, University of South Carolina, presentation to this committee, March 25, 2005.

103. Plato. Phaedrus.

104. J. Macoubrie. 2005. Informed Public Perceptions of Nanotechnology and Trust in Government. Washington, D.C.: Woodrow Wilson International Center for Scholars Project on Emerging Nanotechnologies.

105. J. Macoubrie. 2005. Informed Public Perceptions of Nanotechnology and Trust in Government. Washington, D.C.: Woodrow Wilson International Center for Scholars Project on Emerging Nanotechnologies.

106. See http://www.nanojury.org/, accessed March 2006.

107. Nanotechnology Interdisciplinary Research Team. Undated. From laboratory to society: Developing an informed approach to nanoscale science and technology. Grant 0304448. Nano Science and Technology Studies, University of South Carolina. See http://nsts.nano.sc.edu/nirt.html.

108. A. Laing. 2005. A Report on Canadian and American News Media Coverage of Nano-technology Issues. Comex Research.

109. S.M. Friedman and B.P. Egolf. 2005. Nanotechnology: Risks and the media. IEEE Technology and Society Magazine 24 (Winter):5-11.

110. For example, second-order consequences of improving health and extending life span may include the many social and economic challenges of caring for a larger population of elders.

111. C.M. Cooney. 2006. Some new funding at EPA amid a 4% drop. Environmental Science & Technology Online News. February 22. Available at http://pubs.acs.org/subscribe/journals/esthag-w/2006/feb/policy/cc_newfunding.html, accessed March 2006.

112. Environmental Protection Agency (EPA). 2006. $5 Million awarded to study health and environmental effects of nanotechnology. Press release, March 16. Available at http://yosemite.epa.gov/opa/admpress.nsf/68b5f2d54f3eefd28525701500517fbf/6d536a255f4416848525713300520f80!OpenDocument, accessed March 2006.

113. A.M. Thayer. 2006. Chance of a lifetime. Chemical and Engineering News 84(18):10-18.

5

Molecular Self-Assembly

The National Research Council Committee to Review the National Nano-technology Initiative was asked to "determine the technical feasibility of molecular self-assembly for the manufacture of materials and devices at the molecular scale."[1] The committee convened a workshop of experts in February 2005 to examine the technical information and discuss the issues. With input from the participants, the committee parsed this task into two parts: to consider the technical feasibility of self-assembly first, for the manufacture of materials, and second, for the manufacture of devices. In this system of nomenclature materials are undifferentiated structures. Devices are more complex, with parts or structures dedicated to particular functions. For instance, a lump of brass is a material, while a brass door hardware set has various functional parts (knob, latch, etc.) and is thus a device. A wafer of silicon is a material, while a silicon transistor has various functional parts (electrical contacts, conducting channel, etc.) and is thus a device. Devices typically are made from various materials.

After further discussion, the committee elected to address in addition a broader question—the feasibility of manufacturing systems capable of building, with molecular precision, complex systems that consist of multiple components. The committee's discussions are summarized below, and the workshop agenda is given in Appendix C.

WHAT IS SELF-ASSEMBLY?

In the broadest sense, self-assembly describes the natural tendency of physical systems to exchange energy with their surroundings and assume patterns or structures of reduced free energy. Random thermal motions bring constituent particles together in various configurations, so that stable configurations (those with significant binding energy) form, tend to persist, and eventually become predominant. Through this simple operation of physical law, pattern or structure arises in a bounded system with the input of relatively little information from outside. The information on how to assemble the structure is embodied in the structures of the individual components. A system slowly approaching equilibrium will assume a simple repetitive structure, while a dynamic system may generate structures of great complexity. For example, molecules in a cooling bucket of water will self-assemble as simple ice crystals, while the same molecules in a turbulent cloud with ever-changing temperature and humidity will self-assemble as complex snowflakes in enormous variety. Many fascinating structures in the natural world around us are self-assembled.

Chemists and biologists often use the term self-assembly in a more restricted sense to describe structure formation in a fluid containing various types of molecules, particularly organic molecules that form weak chemical bonds with a strength that depends sensitively on molecular shape and orientation. The strongest bond between such molecules often occurs when the molecules fit together in a "lock and key" fashion. Biological molecules such as proteins are particularly suited to forming complex higher-order structures. For example, the bacterial ribosome—a complex molecular machine consisting of about 55 different protein molecules and several ribosomal RNA molecules—will, under appropriate conditions, self-assemble in a test tube.[2]

MOLECULAR SELF-ASSEMBLY AS A MANUFACTURING TECHNOLOGY

For the Manufacture of Materials

Relatively complex materials such as semi-permeable membranes are manufactured every day by processes that exemplify molecular self-assembly. In a broad sense, fabrication and manufacturing processes for many common materials are exercises in self-assembly—quenching, solidification and crystallization, solution- and vapor-phase chemical reactions, and polymerization. The properties of the resulting materials—for example, the strength of metals or the electron mobility of semiconductors—depend exquisitely on the self-assembly of atoms and molecules to form the atomic and molecular structure of the finished material. The trick for the technologist is to find just the right variation of process conditions—for example, the changes in temperature or the addition of impurities—that result in the desired material properties. Therefore, molecular self-assembly is certainly feasible for the manufacture of materials.

For the Manufacture of Devices

Simple devices such as sensors for medical diagnostics are built every day with the aid of processes that exemplify molecular self-assembly. More complex structures can be generated by more sophisticated self-assembly processes. Processes requiring dynamic steering of process variables are often called "directed" self-assembly. "Templated" self-assembly describes processes requiring control of spatial boundaries such as container material and geometry. Thus, molecular self-assembly is also feasible for the manufacture of devices.

Challenges

As spatial and temporal variations of boundary conditions and process variables become more complex, the emphasis shifts from self-assembly to the flow of information in the control system. However, the committee could not identify a "bright line" distinction between self-assembly and more complex integrated manufacturing processes. For instance, the above-mentioned example of the self-assembly of the bacterial ribosome from its constituent proteins is an elegant biological phenomenon, but it is only one part of the complex process that has evolved to build the ribosome. The various constituent proteins are themselves the product of RNA-driven amino acid catalysis called RNA translation in other functioning ribosomes, and RNA molecules are, in turn, the product of another catalytic process called DNA transcription. This complex assembly process, proceeding in every living cell, involves more than just self-assembly.

Manufacturing processes that can build very complex objects with high yield and repeatability will generally include processes more complex than simple self-assembly. This statement follows primarily from the fact that simple self-assembly does not include a mechanism for error correction.[3] The error rate for assembly of any two constituent parts can often be arranged to be very low, but the total probability of any error will tend to be the sum of the error rates for assembly of all the individual parts. Thus, the probability of a critical error occurring at some point in the assembly process will increase with the complexity of the system and the number of parts that must interoperate. At some level of complexity, the yield of a simple self-assembly process will become negligible.

Practical manufacturing systems solve this problem in a number of ways.

Kinetic constraints on the possible motions of constituents can greatly reduce the error rate in the assembly of constituent parts. Error-correction processes, such as sorting, refining, and purification, can provide a supply of good subcomponents for the next stage in a hierarchical self-assembly. These and other mechanisms are found in engineered manufacturing systems and in the structures and processes of biology.

Thus, the important task before the committee was to assess the feasibility of sophisticated manufacturing processes to produce more complex materials, devices, and, perhaps even entire complex systems from molecular components in a bottom-up fashion. Such processes are not usually considered to be examples of self-assembly.

CURRENT STATE

The current states of two different technologies that have relevance to "bottom-up" or molecular manufacturing are described below. Lithography and nano-biotechnology are very different fields using vastly different methods, and, through the examples they provide, both enlighten the discussion of technical feasibility and future applications.

Microelectronics Manufacturing: Lithography

As scientists and engineers have gained confidence in their ability to develop bottom-up manufacturing processes that exploit the principles of biology, their ability to build small structures "top down" has also rapidly improved. Top-down processes are exemplified by machining, where the desired structure is produced by cutting, drilling, grinding, polishing, or otherwise shaping a block of material. For most of human history, machining was limited to structures that were readily visible to the naked eye. The ability to machine smaller structures developed slowly during the industrial revolution and accelerated with the beginnings of information technology as ever smaller components led to ever faster and more affordable computing, information storage, and communication. Today's microelectronics factories use photolithographic processes to optically project desired structural patterns onto silicon wafers coated with a thin film of photosensitive polymer. After chemical development, the patterned polymer is used as a mask to transfer the desired structure to the silicon, typically by an etching process. In a very real sense, these lithographic systems are the "machine tools" of the information age.

At the time of this writing, the latest generation of microelectronics factories uses 90-nanometer technology, meaning that the lithographic systems and associated etching and deposition processes can routinely build circuits with wires as narrow as 90 nanometers. Certain critical features, such as the transistor gate length, can be even smaller. Pattern dimensions must be controlled to tight tolerances. For example, if the transistor gate length is 40 nanometers, the allowable variance in this dimension (within three standard deviations) would be a few nanometers. This level of precision is necessary because the behavior of each transistor depends sensitively on the gate dimension, and the millions of transistors on a silicon chip cannot interoperate unless each device operates in nearly the same way as the others.

Currently semiconductor manufacturers are equipping the first 65-nanometer factories. In addition, 45- and 32-nanometer manufacturing processes and tools are already under development. At what point will this progression end? Several classes of commercially available lithographic systems—electron beam writers, various contact printing systems, and scanning probe systems—can define structures as small as 5 to 10 nanometers. These systems cannot yet meet the high-volume demands of microelectronics manufacturing, but they are already used in some "niche" manufacturing applications. At the research frontier, scanning probe systems have shown some ability to pattern matter one atom at a time. Many of the experiments involve the comparatively easy placement of metal atoms on atomically smooth metal surfaces. The resulting structures are weakly bonded and only stable at cryogenic temperatures. A few experiments have demonstrated some control of strong covalent bond interactions. For example, Hla and co-workers were able to induce all elementary steps of a simple organic chemical reaction by using various manipulations with a scanning tunneling microscope.[4] An explicitly lithographic process with atomic site specificity is the "hydrogen passivation resist" pioneered by Lyding's group at the University of Illinois in the 1990s.[5] The process involves covering (passivating) a silicon wafer with a single layer of hydrogen atoms and removing selected hydrogen atoms with an electrical current from a scanning probe tip. The hydrogen-silicon bond is stable enough that the resulting pattern can be used to mask further chemical reactions on the surface, with atomic site specificity, at room temperature and above. In 2004, scientists associated with the Australian National Quantum Computer project used this method to introduce single atoms of phosphorus into a silicon crystal at selected atomic sites.[6] In order to perform this feat of atomic-resolution lithography, the silicon surface had to be atomically flat with a low density of defects to allow the formation of a nearly perfect hydrogen resist layer with one hydrogen bond for each surface silicon atom. Desorption of single hydrogen atoms required a scanning probe system equipped with an atomically sharp tungsten tip.

It should be noted that the atomically flat and clean silicon surface, the hydrogen layer, and the atomically sharp tungsten tip were each prepared by simple chemical processes—that is, processes that embody the bottom-up concept of self-assembly. Only the selective removal of single hydrogen atoms embodies the top-down concept of machining. Essentially all of today's practical manufacturing processes mix top-down and bottom-up processes.

These results suggest that there is no fundamental physical barrier to practicing lithography at atomic dimensions. Of course, there is a vast gulf between these slow and very difficult pioneering experiments and today's high-volume, high-yield lithographic manufacturing processes. If the minimum lithographic dimension in large-scale manufacturing continued to be halved roughly every 5 years, atomic-scale lithography would be used in industrial processes in about 40 years. The actual course of technological developments will depend on many factors that cannot be predicted. The silicon transistor, the dominant device of information technology, will not function if shrunk toward atomic dimensions. Economic incentives to continue the current furious pace of research and development in top-down manufacturing might depend on currently unforeseen inventions of new devices that will require or benefit from extreme miniaturization.

Whether or not atomic-resolution lithography can be developed on an industrial scale, there is a rapidly growing body of research results in which lithographic patterns are used as templates to guide the self-assembly of smaller structures. In one recent example, a specially formulated polymer spontaneously forms nanometer-scale patterns that self-align with larger lithographic features, enabling construction of experimental "nanowire" transistors.[7] This is a technique of great interest for fabrication of a variety of next-generation transistor structures. A bit further out, some scientists envision the use of increasingly sophisticated self-assembly processes, including biomolecular processes such as those discussed below, to routinely bridge between the molecular scale and the larger structures that are readily fabricated with the aid of lithography. The result would be the ability to build structures approaching or exceeding biological levels of complexity—a capability that would have enormous implications for information technology, medicine, and energy production, and for endeavors not yet imagined.

Structural Chemistry: Nanobiotechnology

The ability to engineer biological systems has long been a goal of biochemists that has recently been taken up by a new generation of physical scientists. Existing work on recombinant DNA molecules holds promise for the construction and evaluation of new gene arrangements.[8] The new applications of nanotechnological techniques to biological systems hold substantial promise.[9] Today, rudimentary devices have been produced, including sensors and actuators, input and output devices, and genetic circuits to control cells.[10] Future developments in this new structural chemistry will target both the stabilization and the simulation of biomolecules for use in a wide range of activities, including various manufacturing processes.

A number of strategies have been demonstrated by which the material properties of biomolecular systems may be moved outside the relatively constrained environment of the living cell. Perhaps the simplest example is the direct substitution of nonbiological organic or inorganic chemistries for bioorganic chemistries. Examples include bacteria grown in extreme environments and enzymes that catalyze reactions at high pressures and temperatures found outside the normal range of conditions for life processes. The protein complex responsible for production of oxygen in photosynthesis does not, in fact, operate in an aqueous environment but in an electrochemical interphase region of complex physical chemistry including an extremely high electric field, greater than 20 megavolts per meter.[11] Once the structure and the function of a specific biomolecule are elucidated, it should be possible in many cases to simply substitute alternative forms of chemistry for selected components. Protein engineering is already addressing this strategy in a rudimentary manner in synthetic amino acid analogs. Preliminary experimental validation that such nanobiotechnology may be useful for manufacturing is found in the ability to design synthetic bis-amino acid oligomers to have specific rigid shapes, which should be useful in constructing complex atomically precise three-dimensional objects.[12]

Fully synthetic analogs can be created today by molecular imprinting, a technique to create template-shaped cavities in polymer matrices with memory of the template molecules. This technique is based on the system used by natural enzymes for substrate recognition, which is called the "lock and key" model. In recent decades, the molecular imprinting technique has been developed for use in receptors, chromatographic separations, catalysis, and fine chemical sensing.[13] Structural biologists can now engineer enzymes to interact with chemicals that do not occur in nature. For example, proteins have been modified to bind poison gas and explosives so that they can be used as single-molecule sensors, and motor proteins have been modified from their natural function and show promise as mechanical components in hybrid nano-engineered systems. In one such system, the cytoplasmic fragment of the F1-ATPase has been integrated into self-assembled nanomechanical systems as a mechanical actuator.[14] Repeated cycles of zinc addition and removal by chelation result in inhibition and restoration, respectively, of motor rotation in the engineered protein. These results demonstrate the ability to engineer single-molecule chemical regulation into a biomolecular motor. Using these methods, synthetic biologists eventually aim to build cells from the ground up rather than tinkering with a handful of genes or tweaking a metabolic pathway or two, as do today's genetic engineers.

A third strategy is the stabilization of biomolecules in biomolecular-materials composites. For example, nanoporous materials can be specifically tailored to accommodate individual protein catalysts. Such materials could simultaneously protect the bulk protein molecule from destructive physical forces while retaining a channel to the catalytic site. The ability to synthesize biological macromolecules with novel materials components creates both the opportunity to build enzymes that function outside the normal cellular environment and the opportunity to modify the cellular environment by filling it with hybrid biomolecular-materials composites. The synthesis of DNA molecules containing metallo-base pairs creates a molecular structure that can transfer both biological information and an electrical signal. Methodology has recently been developed to genetically encode novel amino acids. This has already been used to create heavy-atom-containing amino acids to facilitate x-ray crystallographic studies; amino acids with novel steric/packing and electronic properties; photocrosslinking amino acids that can be used to probe protein-protein interactions in vitro or in vivo; and keto- and acetylene-containing amino acids that can be used to selectively introduce a large number of biophysical probes, tags, and novel chemical functions.[15]

As the examples above make clear, the lines between nanotechnology and biotechnology are becoming blurred. Indeed, at the molecular level of structure, the border between living and nonliving materials is also rapidly fading. This reality begins to redefine commonly used definitions and confounds accepted paradigms.

Technical Feasibility of Site-Specific Chemistry for Large-Scale Manufacturing

Prudent extrapolation of the current research results presented above suggests an amazing future for nanotechnology. Indeed, many scientists foresee a long-term future in which a variety of strategies, tools, and processes allow nearly any stable chemical structure to be built atom by atom or molecule by molecule from the bottom up. However, there is still a gulf between this vision and popular images of nanotechnology in which the bottom-up approach is routinely used to manufacture complex, large-scale industrial objects such as computers or buildings at very low cost. The feasibility of such developments would depend on the attainable *efficiency* of the manufacturing processes. The proposed manufacturing systems[16–19] can be viewed as highly miniaturized, highly articulated versions of today's scanning probe systems, or perhaps as engineered ribosome-like systems designed to assemble a wide range of molecular building blocks in two or three dimensions rather than the linear assembly of amino acids by the ribosome. In this approach, reactions are described with both reagent and product as part of extended "handle" structures, which can be moved mechanically.[20] To be practical for the manufacture of large-scale objects, such mechanisms would have to operate at a very low error rate, a very high speed, and near-perfect thermodynamic efficiency. Technical arguments for the eventual attainability of these attributes have been provided.[21] Design strategies have been outlined that, it is maintained, would allow such systems to greatly exceed the error rates, speed, and average thermodynamic efficiency of naturally evolved biological systems. Proponents of these design and manufacturing strategies foresee the exploitation of exquisitely controlled site-specific chemistry on a vast industrial scale. While scanning probe systems have demonstrated the feasibility of some site-specific reactions, scale-up to manufacturing systems is still a daunting task, and the majority of nanoscale scientists and engineers believe it is too early to try to predict the ultimate capabilities of such systems.

The committee found the evaluation of the feasibility of these ideas to be difficult because of the lack of experimental demonstrations of many of the key underlying concepts. The technical arguments make use of accepted scientific knowledge but constitute a "theoretical analysis demonstrating the possibility of a class of as-yet *unrealizable* devices."[22] Thus, this work is currently outside the mainstream of both conventional science (designed to seek new knowledge) and conventional engineering (usually concerned with the design of things that can be built more or less immediately). Rather, it may be in the tradition of visionary engineering analysis exemplified by Konstantin Tsiolkovski's 1903 publication, "The Exploration of Cosmic Space by Means of Reaction Devices,"[23] and today's studies of "space elevators" based on hypothetical carbon nanotube composite materials.[24]

Construction of extended structures with three-dimensional covalent bonding may be easy to conceive and might be readily accomplished, but only by using tools that do not yet exist.[25] In other words, the tool structures and other components cannot yet be built, but they can be computationally modeled. Modeling the thermodynamic stability of a structure (showing that it can, in principle, exist) does not tell one how to build it, and these arguments do not yet constitute a research strategy or a research plan.

To bring this field forward, meaningful connections are needed between the relevant scientific communities. Examples include:

- Delineating desirable research directions not already being pursued by the biochemistry community;
- Defining and focusing on some basic experimental steps that are critical to advancing long-term goals; and
- Outlining some "proof-of-principle" studies that, if successful, would provide knowledge or engineering demonstrations of key principles or components with immediate value.

CONCLUSIONS

Materials and devices of moderate complexity can be designed and manufactured by molecular self-assembly. Although self-assembly operates on simple and well-understood scientific principles, understanding of the details is far from complete. The ultimate potential of self-assembly processes in nature and in engineered manufacturing systems remains to be explored.

Proceeding beyond simple self-assembly, there is experimental evidence that biological systems can be modified to operate in conditions far outside those of the living cell, and therefore, many biotechnologists believe that these systems will form the basis for many future manufacturing processes.[26] Manufacturing trends and research directions in information technology and related fields also suggest the eventual development of manufacturing processes with some capability to pattern structures with atomic precision.[27]

Although theoretical calculations can be made today, the eventually attainable range of chemical reaction cycles, error rates, speed of operation, and thermodynamic efficiencies of such bottom-up manufacturing systems cannot be reliably predicted at this time. Thus, the eventually attainable perfection and complexity of manufactured products, while they can be calculated in theory, cannot be predicted with confidence. Finally, the optimum research paths that might lead to systems which greatly exceed the thermodynamic efficiencies and other capabilities of biological systems cannot be reliably predicted at this time. Research funding that is based on the ability of investigators to produce experimental demonstrations that link to abstract models and guide long-term vision is most appropriate to achieve this goal.

NOTES

1. U.S. Congress. Public Law 108-153. 2003. 21st Century Nanotechnology Research and Development Act. 15 USC 7501. 108 Cong., December 3.
2. B. Alberts, D. Bray, J. Lewis, M. Raff, K. Roberts, and J.D. Watson. 1994. Molecular Biology of the Cell. Third Edition. New York: Garland Publishing.
3. To be more precise, at a given temperature and with a given set of constituents, there is no mechanism to reduce the error rate below a level inherent in the random thermal motions that facilitate the assembly. The error rate may be reduced by reducing the temperature, but this quickly leads to an unacceptably slow assembly process. The error rate can also be reduced by using a small number of very distinct constituents so that error states involve a large increase in the free energy of the system.
4. S.W. Hla, L. Bartels, G. Meyer, and K.H. Rieder. 2000. Inducing all steps of a chemical reaction with the scanning tunneling microscope tip: Towards single molecule engineering. Phys. Rev. Lett. 85:2777.
5. J.W. Lyding, T.-C. Shen, J.S. Hubacek, J.R. Tucker, and G.C. Abeln. 1994. Nanoscale patterning and oxidation of H-passivated Si(100)-2×1 surfaces with an ultrahigh vacuum scanning tunneling microscope. Appl. Phys. Lett. 64:2010.

6. S.R. Schofield, N.J. Curson, M.Y. Simmons, F.J. Rueß, T. Hallam, L. Oberbeck, and R.G. Clark. 2003. Atomically precise placement of single dopants in Si. Phys. Rev. Lett. 91:136104.
7. C.T. Black. 2005. Self-aligned self-assembly of multi-nanowire silicon field effect transistors. Appl. Phys. Lett. 87:163116.
8. W. Szybalski and A. Skalka. 1978 Nobel prizes and restriction enzymes. Gene 4:181-182.
9. A. Matouschek and C. Bustamante. 2003. Finding a protein's Achilles heel. Nat. Struct. Biol. 10(9):674-676.
10. D. Ferber. 2004. Synthetic biology: Microbes made to order. Science 303:158-161.
11. K.N. Ferreira, T.M. Iverson, K. Maghlaoui, J. Barber, and S. Iwata. 2004. Architecture of the photosynthetic oxygen-evolving center. Science 303:1831-1838.
12. S. Pornsuwan, C.E. Schafmeister, and S. Saxena. 2006. Flexibility and lengths of bis-peptide nanostructures by electron spin resonance. J. Am. Chem. Soc. Accepted for publication.
13. A.J. Hall, M. Emgenbroich, and B. Sellergren. 2005. Imprinted polymers. Topics in Current Chemistry 249:317-349.
14. H. Liu, J.J. Schmidt, G.D. Bachand, S.S. Rizk, L.L. Looger, H.W. Hellinga, and C.D. Montemagno. 2002. Control of a biomolecular motor-powered nanodevice with an engineered chemical switch. Nat. Mater. 1(3):173-177.
15. P. Schulz. 2005. Synthesis at the Interface of Chemistry and Biology. Available at http://schultz.scripps.edu/research.html, accessed March 2006.
16. K.E. Drexler. 1981. Molecular engineering: An approach to the development of general capabilities for molecular manipulation. Proceedings of the National Academy of Sciences 78:5275.
17. K.E. Drexler. 1986. Engines of Creation. New York: Anchor Press/Doubleday.
18. K.E. Drexler. 1992. Nanosystems, Molecular Machinery, Manufacturing and Computation. New York: Wiley & Sons.
19. D.S. Goodsell. 2004. Bionanotechnology: Lessons from Nature. New York: Wiley & Sons.
20. K.E. Drexler. 1992. Nanosystems, Molecular Machinery, Manufacturing and Computation. New York: Wiley & Sons.
21. K.E. Drexler. 1992. Nanosystems, Molecular Machinery, Manufacturing and Computation. New York: Wiley & Sons.
22. K.E. Drexler. 1992. Nanosystems, Molecular Machinery, Manufacturing and Computation. New York: Wiley & Sons.
23. K.E. Tsiolkovski. 1903. The exploration of cosmic space by means of reaction devices. (Issledovanie mirovykh prostranstv reaktivuymi priboram.) Nauchnoe Obozrenie, No. 5. St. Petersburg, Russia.
24. B.C. Edwards. 2005. A hoist to the heavens. IEEE Spectrum Online 36. Available at http://www.spectrum.ieee.org/aug05/1690, accessed March 2006.
25. M. Rieth and W. Schommers, eds. 2005. Handbook of Computational and Theoretical Nanotechnology. American Scientific Publishers.
26. See in this chapter the subsection titled "Structural Chemistry: Nanobiotechnology."
27. See in this chapter the subsection titled "Microelectronics Manufacturing: Lithography."

Appendixes

A

Statement of Task

In response to a directive from the U.S. Congress, the National Research Council established the Committee to Review the National Nanotechnology Initiative. The task to be addressed by the committee was set forth in the 21st Century Nanotechnology Research and Development Act, Section 5, Public Law 108-153,[1] as follows:

Triennial External Review of the National Nanotechnology Program.

(a) IN GENERAL—The Director of the National Nanotechnology Coordination Office shall enter into an arrangement with the National Research Council of the National Academy of Sciences to conduct a triennial evaluation of the Program, including—

    (1) an evaluation of the technical accomplishments of the Program, including a review of whether the Program has achieved the goals under the metrics established by the Council;

    (2) A review of the Program's management and coordination across agencies and disciplines;

    (3) A review of the funding levels at each agency for the Program's activities and the ability of each agency to achieve the Program's stated goals with that funding;

    (4) An evaluation of the Program's success in transferring technology to the private sector;

    (5) An evaluation of whether the Program has been successful in fostering interdisciplinary research and development;

---

[1] U.S. Congress. 2003. 21st Century Nanotechnology Research and Development Act. Public Law 108-153. 15 USC 7501. 108 Cong., December 3.

(6) An evaluation of the extent to which the Program has adequately considered ethical, legal, environmental, and other appropriate societal concerns;

(7) Recommendations for new or revised Program goals;

(8) Recommendations for new research areas, partnerships, coordination and management mechanisms, or programs to be established to achieve the Program's stated goals;

(9) Recommendations on policy, program, and budget changes with respect to nanotechnology research and development activities;

(10) Recommendations for improved metrics to evaluate the success of the Program in accomplishing its stated goals;

(11) A review of the performance of the National Nanotechnology Coordination Office and its efforts to promote access to and early application of the technologies, innovations, and expertise derived from Program activities to agency missions and systems across the Federal Government and to United States industry;

(12) An analysis of the relative position of the United States compared to other nations with respect to nanotechnology research and development, including the identification of any critical research areas where the United States should be the world leader to best achieve the goals of the Program; and

(13) An analysis of the current impact of nanotechnology on the United States economy and recommendations for increasing its future impact.

(b) STUDY ON MOLECULAR SELF-ASSEMBLY.—As part of the first triennial review conducted in accordance with subsection (a), the National Research Council shall conduct a one-time study to determine the technical feasibility of molecular self-assembly for the manufacture of materials and devices at the molecular scale.

(c) STUDY ON THE RESPONSIBLE DEVELOPMENT OF NANOTECHNOLOGY.—As part of the first triennial review conducted in accordance with subsection (a), the National Research Council shall conduct a one-time study to assess the need for standards, guidelines, or strategies for ensuring the responsible development of nanotechnology, including, but not limited to—

(1) Self-replicating nanoscale machines or devices;

(2) The release of such machines in natural environments;

(3) Encryption;

(4) The development of defensive technologies;

(5) The use of nanotechnology in the enhancement of human intelligence; and

(6) The use of nanotechnology in developing artificial intelligence.

B

Committee Biographies

James C. Williams, *Chair*, NAE, is professor of materials science and engineering and Honda Chair at the Ohio State University (OSU). He is a member of the National Academy of Engineering, a fellow of ASM International, a fellow of TMS-AIME, and a former member of the Air Force Scientific Advisory Board. He was the ASM/TMS Distinguished Lecturer in Materials and Society in 1997, and the ASM Campbell Lecturer in 1999. Dr. Williams' research has focused on phase transformations, processing, and structure-property relations in high-performance materials, mainly Ti, Ni, and Al alloys. He has also been extensively involved in technology policy related to materials. Before OSU, Dr. Williams held research and leadership positions at General Electric, Boeing, and Rockwell. He also spent 13 years at Carnegie Mellon University, where he was a professor, president of the Mellon Institute, and dean of engineering. He is regularly invited to lecture at meetings and conferences both in the United States and abroad. Dr. Williams has published over 200 papers based on his research, is the editor of the three-volume proceedings of the 1976 International Titanium Conference, held in Moscow, and holds two patents. In addition, he served as commissioner on the National Research Council's Commission for Engineering and Technical Systems, as well as chair of the Los Alamos National Laboratory's Division Review Committee, Materials Science and Technology. He has received the ASM Gold Medal Award (1992), the TMS Leadership Award (1993), and the Spirit Award, Prairie View A&M University (1994), in addition to the Distinguished Engineering Alumnus Award (1992) and the College of Engineering Distinguished Lecturer Award (1999), both from the

University of Washington. Dr. Williams received a Ph.D. from the University of Washington in 1968.

Cherry A. Murray, *Vice Chair,* NAS, NAE, is the Deputy Director for Science and Technology (DDST) at Lawrence Livermore National Laboratory. Murray is a physicist who has been nationally recognized for her work in surface physics, light scattering, and complex fluids. She is a member of the National Academy of Sciences, the National Academy of Engineering, and the American Academy of Arts and Sciences. As the DDST, Murray leads and oversees the laboratory's multidisciplinary science and technology activities, including the laboratory's $110 million institutional research and development program. Murray, formerly senior vice president for Physical Sciences and Wireless Research at Bell Labs Lucent Technologies, first joined Bell Labs in 1978 and held a number of Bell Lab research and management positions. In 2000, Murray became vice president for Physical Sciences and then senior vice president in 2001. In this role, Murray managed the wireless, nanotechnology, and physical research laboratories and was chair of the New Jersey Nanotechnology Consortium. Murray received her B.S. and Ph.D. in physics from the Massachusetts Institute of Technology. She serves on the governing boards of the National Research Council and Argonne National Laboratory. She is the recipient of numerous awards, and *Discover Magazine* named her one of the "50 Most Important Women in Science" in 2002.

A. Michael Andrews II is vice president and chief technology officer at L-3 Communications, reporting to the chairman and chief executive officer. He guides the company's long-term R&D initiatives, provides input on new solutions to DOD requirements, and continually evaluates the evolving technologies used in L-3 products. Before that, he served as deputy assistant secretary of research and technology and chief scientist for the United States Army, a position he held since 1998. Dr. Andrews' effective work with senior staff principals, scientists, and engineers from the Army, DOD, and industry significantly enhanced the Army's efforts to develop the Future Combat Systems, Objective Force, and Force Transformation. Prior to joining the Army in 1997, Dr. Andrews held a variety of corporate engineering leadership and system development positions at Rockwell International. He began his career at Rockwell in 1971, working on electro-optic and infrared research and development products. An author of over 50 technical articles, Dr. Andrews holds several patents in infrared sensors, materials, and signal processors. He is a recipient of various honors, including the Presidential Rank Award, the Meritorious Civilian Service Award, Rockwell's Engineer of the Year Award, and the University of Illinois Distinguished Alumnus Award and is a fellow of the Institute of Electrical and Electronics Engineers. Dr. Andrews received his

B.S. and M.S. in electrical engineering from the University of Oklahoma and his Ph.D. in electrical engineering from the University of Illinois.

Mark J. Cardillo is the executive director of the Camille and Henry Dreyfus Foundation. Dr. Cardillo received his B.S. from the Stevens Institute of Technology in 1964 and his Ph.D. in chemistry from Cornell University in 1970. He served as a research associate at Brown University, a CNR research scientist at the University of Genoa, and a PRF research fellow in the mechanical engineering department at the Massachusetts Institute of Technology. In 1975, Dr. Cardillo joined Bell Laboratories as a member of the technical staff in the surface physics department. He was appointed head of the chemical physics research department in 1981 and subsequently named head of the photonics materials research department. Most recently, he was director of broadband access research. Dr. Cardillo is a fellow of the American Physical Society. He has been the Phillips Lecturer at Haverford College and a Langmuir Lecturer of the American Chemical Society. He received the Medard Welch Award of the American Vacuum Society in 1987, the Innovations in Real Materials Award in 1998, and the Pel Associates Award in Applied Polymer Chemistry in 2000.

Crystal Cunanan is vice president for development and operations at ReVision Optics, Inc. Previously, she was director of tissue engineering at Arbor Surgical Technologies, Inc., following her tenure as manager of the biosciences group at Edwards Lifesciences Corporation. She has over 20 years of industrial experience in permanently implanted devices. Her research has focused on all modes of interaction between biomedical devices and the body. Specific topics have included the chemistry, design, testing, and qualification of polymeric and biopolymeric implant materials, such as silicones, silicone copolymers, acrylates, hydrogels, collages, and hyaluronic acid; the development of new in vivo and in vitro models to study material-biological interactions, such as cell adhesion, migration, toxicity, and wound healing; and the characterization of material surfaces and the characterization's relationship to biological reactions. Ms. Cunanan holds 26 issued U.S. patents and published applications and is the author of over 40 papers, presentations, and published abstracts. She is active in several professional societies and serves on the board of the Healthcare Businesswoman's Association. She is the chair of the National Academies roundtable discussion group on Biomedical Engineered Materials and Applications and has served as chair of the industrial advisory board committee of the University of Washington Engineered Biomaterials (UWEB) Engineering Research Center. Ms. Cunanan received a B.S. in biology and a B.S. in chemistry from the University of California, Irvine, in 1982, and an M.S. in chemistry from the University of California, San Diego, in 1984. In 2004,

Ms. Cunanan was awarded a certificate in bioinformatics by the California State University, Fullerton.

Peter H. Diamandis is the chair, founder, and president of the X Prize Foundation, a nonprofit organization promoting the formation of a space-tourism industry by offering a $10 million prize. Dr. Diamandis is also founder, chair, and CEO of Zero Gravity Corporation, a commercial space company developing private, FAA-certified parabolic flight utilizing Boeing 727-200 aircraft. He was a co-founder of Space Adventures, as well as a co-founder and chair of Starport.com, a leading Internet site for space exploration, which was acquired by SPACE.com in 1990. In 1987, Dr. Diamandis co-founded the International Space University (ISU), where he served as the university's first program director and trustee. Before that, Dr. Diamandis served as chair of Students for the Exploration and Development of Space (SEDS), an organization he founded at the Massachusetts Institute of Technology (MIT) in 1980. Dr. Diamandis received his undergraduate and graduate degrees in aerospace engineering from MIT and his M.D. from Harvard Medical School. He has conducted research in a number of fields, including molecular genetics, space medicine, and launch vehicle design. Dr. Diamandis has received a number of awards, including MIT's Kresge Award, the 1986 Space Industrialization Fellowship, the 1988 Aviation Week & Space Technology Laurel, the 1993 Space Frontier Pioneer Award, and the Russian 1995 K.E. Tsiolkovsky Award.

Paul A. Fleury, NAS, NAE, is dean of engineering at Yale University, where he also serves as the Frederick W. Beinecke Professor of Engineering and of Applied Physics and as a professor of physics. His primary research interests lie in materials performance and properties as revealed by modern probes such as lasers, neutrons, and synchrotron light sources. Dr. Fleury joined Yale after 4 years as the dean of engineering at the University of New Mexico. Prior to that, he worked at AT&T Bell Laboratories in Murray Hill, New Jersey, for 30 years, serving as director of materials and processing research. In 1992-1993, Dr. Fleury was vice president of research and exploratory technologies at Sandia National Laboratories. He has published more than 130 technical papers in scientific books and journals and holds five patents on optical and electro-optical devices. Dr. Fleury is a fellow of the American Physical Society and the American Association for the Advancement of Science, as well as a member of the American Society for Engineering Education and the Connecticut Academy of Science and Engineering. He is the recipient of the Frank Isakson Prize of the American Physical Society and the Michelson Morley Award. Dr. Fleury received B.S. and M.S. degrees in physics at John Carroll University in 1960 and 1962, respectively. He earned his Ph.D. in physics from the Massachusetts Institute of Technology in 1965. He was awarded the SRC Senior

Visiting Fellowship at Oxford University, as well as a National Science Foundation graduate fellowship. Dr. Fleury is a member of Sigma Xi and Tau Beta Pi.

Paul B. Germeraad is the founder and president of Intellectual Assets, Inc., a professional advisory services firm specializing in integrated business, research and development, and intellectual property processes. His past roles include chief operating officer for Aurigin Systems, Inc., where he focused on the development of the company's intellectual asset management products for the competitive intelligence, licensing, and R&D communities. Prior to joining Aurigin in 1998, Dr. Germeraad served as vice president of corporate research for Avery Dennison, where he directed the company's corporate research center. Before joining Avery Dennison, Dr. Germeraad held a variety of R&D and management positions at Raychem Corporation and was director of James River Corporation's Flexible Packaging Technical Center. Dr. Germeraad is a graduate of the University of California, San Diego, with a B.A. in chemistry. In addition, he holds a Ph.D. in chemistry from the University of California, Irvine, and an L.L.B. from La Salle University in Chicago. Dr. Germeraad is a past chairman of the board of the Industrial Research Institute, an organization of approximately 300 chief technology officers whose organizations account for over 70 percent of all U.S. R&D spending. Dr. Germeraad holds 10 U.S. patents and 12 foreign counterparts, is a contributing author to two books, and is the author of over a dozen refereed articles.

Alan H. Goldstein is the Fierer Chair and director of the program in biomedical materials engineering science at Alfred University. The university has been a member of NSF's Industry-University Center for Biosurfaces (IUCB) and has received support from the Keck Foundation to establish a center for bioceramic interfacing. Dr. Goldstein has been a member of the Biomedical Engineering Materials and Applications (BEMA) roundtable, a shared activity of the IOM, NAE, and NRC. Through his continuing participation in BEMA, Dr. Goldstein is working to define the key issues at the cutting edge of biomaterials engineering, with a special focus on the coming integration of biomolecules with nonliving materials. He has proposed that this area, which he has termed biomolecular-materials composites, will create both the most useful physical systems and the most challenging bioethical situations at the interface between bioengineering and nanotechnology. In 2003, Dr. Goldstein's work in the bioethics area received international recognition in the form of a Shell-Economist Award for his essay on the topic of nature versus nanoengineering. Dr. Goldstein's research focuses on topics ranging from protein engineering to biomaterials, and he is considered the world's foremost expert on bacterial biodegradation of mineral phosphates. Prior to joining the faculty at Alfred, Dr. Goldstein was a professor at California State University, Los Angeles and at the University of Arizona and was a research scientist at Chevron. He received his Ph.D. in genetics and physical chemistry from the University of Arizona.

Mary L. Good, NAE, is the Donaghey University Professor and dean of the Donaghey College of Information Science and Systems Engineering at the University of Arkansas, Little Rock. Previously Dr. Good served for 4 years as the under secretary for technology for the Technology Administration in the Department of Commerce, a presidentially appointed, Senate-confirmed position. In addition to her role as under secretary for technology, Dr. Good chaired the National Science and Technology Council's Committee on Technological Innovation (NSTC/CTI) and served on the NSTC Committee on National Security. Before joining the administration, Dr. Good was the senior vice president of technology at Allied Signal, Inc., where she was responsible for centralized research and technology organizations. She was a member of the management committee and responsible for technology transfer and commercialization support for new technologies. This position followed assignments as president of Allied Signal's Engineered Material Research Center, director of the UOP Research Center, and president of the Signal Research Center. Before her various positions in industrial research management, Dr. Good spent more than 25 years as a teacher and researcher in the Louisiana State University system. Dr. Good was appointed to the National Science Board by President Carter in 1980 and again by President Reagan in 1986. She was chairman of that board from 1988 until 1991, when she received an appointment from President Bush to become a member of the President's Council of Advisors on Science and Technology (PCAST). Dr. Good also serves as the managing member for Venture Capital Investors, LLC, and on the boards of Biogen in Cambridge, Massachusetts; of IDEXX Laboratories in Westbrook, Maine; and of Acxiom Board in Little Rock, Arkansas. In addition, Dr. Good has served on the boards of Rensselaer Polytechnic Institute, Cincinnati Milacron, and Ameritech. She was also a member of the National Advisory Board for the state of Arkansas. Dr. Good received her B.S. in chemistry from the University of Central Arkansas and her M.S. and Ph.D. in inorganic chemistry from the University of Arkansas. She has also received numerous awards and honorary degrees from many colleges and universities, including, most recently, the College of William and Mary, Polytechnic University of New York, Louisiana State University, and Michigan State University.

Thomas S. Hartwick is retired from general management in the aerospace industry. He has more than 45 years of research and development, technology transfer/insertion, and mainstream business experience supporting all segments of the U.S. government. Dr. Hartwick previously worked at Hughes Aircraft Company, Aerospace Corporation, and TRW. General management positions include electro-optic R&D laboratories, chip R&D and manufacturing, corporate strategic planning, a commercial chip company, and a major satellite payload program. His areas of published research include sensors and imaging, optical communications, magnetic materials, microwave devices, molecular lasers, far-infrared lasers and their applications, and laser heterodyne radiometry. Since leaving the aerospace industry in 1995, Dr. Hartwick has served on a number of academic, government, and industry boards in a technical management role. He is chair (emeritus) of the Advisory Group on Electron Devices in the Office of the Secretary of Defense, chair of NRC committees on aviation security R&D, active with the Defense Science Board and GAO, and active for two decades with the National Technology Transfer Center. He currently serves on five corporate boards/committees and on four government committees. Dr. Hartwick received his Ph.D. in electrical engineering from the University of Southern California, his M.S. in physics from UCLA, and his B.S. in physics from the University of Illinois.

Maynard A. Holliday is a director at Evolution Robotics, a multinational operating company of Idealab that develops robotics solutions and partners with manufacturers to integrate those technologies into intelligent devices for commercial and consumer use. Over the past 20 years, his notable work experience has included robots for use at the Chernobyl disaster site and he was twice named a finalist for the U.S. astronaut corps. Mr. Holliday has managed interdisciplinary projects of international and commercial importance at Lawrence Livermore National Laboratory and at Schlumberger Semiconductor Solutions in Silicon Valley. He was awarded the AAAS Science Engineering and Diplomacy Fellowship in 1995-1996, bringing him to Washington, D.C., to work on technology policy at the U.S. State Department and the Department of Energy (DOE). In 1996, Mr. Holliday assembled and led the joint DOE/NASA International Pioneer Project team that designed and fabricated a radiation-hardened telerobotic mobile vehicle for site characterization and remediation tasks at Chernobyl Unit 4. While at DOE he was awarded the Meritorious Service award, its highest, for his work on the bilateral U.S.–Russian Nuclear Material Security Task Force. Mr. Holliday holds an M.S. in mechanical engineering design from Stanford University, where he focused on robotics, international security, and arms control. He also holds a B.S. in mechanical engineering from Carnegie Mellon University.

Richard L. Irving has served in pastoral positions for communities in California for over 20 years. Since 1997, he has filled the role of senior pastor for the Lakewood Village Community Church in Long Beach, California. Previously, he served for 15 years as the pastor of the First Congregational Church of Santa Ana and for 2 years as the associate pastor for the Community Church of Corona Del

Mar. Rev. Irving received his M.Div. from the Claremont School of Theology in 1980. He has pastoral standing with the National Association of Congregational Christian Churches, the International Council of Community Churches, and the United Church of Christ. Rev. Irving also serves as a community representative on the Edwards Healthcare Animal Care and Use Committee. Prior to pursuing his theological studies, Rev. Irving served for over 5 years as a member of the U.S. Air Force. He commenced military service as an aircraft maintenance officer with the Air Force, with the rank of captain, after receiving his B.A. from California State University, Fullerton. Then, after receiving an M.A. from that same institution, Rev. Irving worked as a program analyst trainee for the Space and Missile Systems Organization of the Air Force.

Donald H. Levy, NAS, is the Albert A. Michelson Distinguished Service Professor in the University of Chicago's James Franck Institute, Department of Chemistry and Physical Sciences Collegiate Division. His current research involves laser spectroscopy in supersonic molecular beams. During his 37-year tenure with the University of Chicago, Dr. Levy has been an Alfred P. Sloan Fellow, a DuPont Faculty Fellow, a John Simon Guggenheim Fellow, and the Ralph and Mary Otis Isham Professor. Before that Dr. Levy spent 3 years at Cambridge University under NIH and NATO postdoctoral fellowships. He received his B.A. from Harvard University in 1961 and his Ph.D. from the University of California, Berkeley, in 1965. Dr. Levy is a fellow of the American Physical Society, the American Association for the Advancement of Science, and the American Academy of Arts and Sciences. He is the recipient of the Plyler Prize of the American Physical Society and the Optical Society of America's Ellis R. Lippincott Award. In addition to the Lady Davis Visiting Professorship at the Technion, Dr. Levy's lectureships include appointments as the Bourke Lecturer, Faraday Division, Royal Society of Chemistry; the Jeremy Musher Memorial Lecturer, Hebrew University; the Albert Noyes Lecturer, Kansas State University; the Frontiers in Chemistry Research Lecturer, Texas A&M University; and the Sigma Xi National Lecturer from 1981 to 1983. Dr. Levy has also served as editor of the *Journal of Chemical Physics* since 1998.

Bettie Sue Siler Masters, IOM, is the Robert A. Welch Foundation Distinguished Professor in Chemistry in the Department of Biochemistry at the University of Texas Health Science Center at San Antonio. She earned her B.S. in chemistry from Roanoke College and her Ph.D. in biochemistry from Duke University. Dr. Masters served as professor and chair of the Department of Biochemistry at the Medical College of Wisconsin, Milwaukee, and professor of biochemistry at the University of Texas Southwestern Medical School at Dallas. She is the recipient of the Bernard B. Brodie Award from the American Society for Pharmacology and Experimental

Therapeutics and the Excellence in Science Award from the Federation of American Societies for Experimental Biology (FASEB). She is a past member of the board of directors and former vice president for science policy of FASEB. Dr. Masters recently completed a 2-year term as president of the American Society for Biochemistry and Molecular Biology. Her research focuses on the structure-function relationships of flavoproteins and heme proteins involved in the production of lipid mediators (fatty acid, prostaglandin, and arachidonic acid metabolites) by cytochromes P450 and of nitric oxide by three isoforms of nitric oxide synthase.

Sonia E. Miller is an attorney admitted to practice in New York and the District of Columbia, before the Supreme Court of the United States, and before the U.S. District Courts of the Southern and Eastern Districts. Ms. Miller's firm, S.E. Miller Law Firm, is dedicated to advising and consulting individuals, industry, government agencies, and nongovernmental organizations, as well as policy makers, educators, and the legal and judicial system in understanding and navigating through the cutting-edge legal, business, ethical, policy, legislative, and regulatory interrelated issues found within emerging and converging technologies such as nanotechnology and nanoscience, biotechnology and genetic engineering, information technology, cognitive science, neuroscience, and other related sciences and technologies. Additionally, Ms. Miller is involved in issues related to human-computer interaction and brain-machine interface. Ms. Miller is founder and global president of the Converging Technologies Bar Association; an adjunct professor in the Executive MBA Program at the Institute for Technology and Enterprise at Polytechnic University in Manhattan, creating and teaching the first university-level class on converging technologies ("Managing Converging Technologies: Integrating Bits, Atoms, Neurons, and Genes"); a columnist on converging technologies for the *New York Law Journal*; and a worldwide solicited speaker and author. She received an M.B.A. in international business and M.S.Ed. and B.Ed. degrees from the University of Miami, and a J.D. from New York Law School.

Edward K. Moran is director of the Tri-State Product Innovation Practice of Deloitte & Touche's Technology, Media & Telecommunications (TMT) group. He also heads up Deloitte's Nanotech Industry Practice and is a leader of its Tri-State VC-backed company practice. Mr. Moran provides TMT clients with consultative assistance in securing financing, strategic planning, product innovation, market segmentation, competitive positioning, and industry analysis. As part of the product innovation process, he also assists TMT clients with the identification of strategic partners and consults on the management of these relationships. Mr. Moran is also executive director of the New York State NanoBusiness Alliance. Prior to joining Deloitte & Touche, he was managing partner of a Manhattan law firm, where he served a number of technology and entertainment clients. He also cofounded a multi-disciplinary consultancy that targeted high-tech and entertainment companies and was a managing director of a Manhattan investment and advisory company that specializes in technology and media investments. Mr. Moran holds a law degree from New York Law School, has an M.B.A. in information systems and in management from New York University, and teaches corporate finance at New York University. He speaks widely on the topics of product innovation, business strategy, nanotechnology, technology transfer, and the financing of technology companies.

David C. Mowery is the William A. and Betty H. Hasler Professor of New Enterprise Development at the Walter A. Haas School of Business at the University of California, Berkeley, a research associate of the National Bureau of Economic Research, and during the 2003-2004 academic year was the Bower Fellow at the Harvard Business School. He received his undergraduate and Ph.D. degrees in economics from Stanford University and was a postdoctoral fellow at the Harvard Business School. Dr. Mowery taught at Carnegie Mellon University, worked as a staff officer for the National Academies, and served in the Office of the United States Trade Representative as a Council on Foreign Relations' International Affairs Fellow. He has been a member of a number of NRC committees, including those on the Competitive Status of the U.S. Civil Aviation Industry, on the Causes and Consequences of the Internationalization of U.S. Manufacturing, on the Federal Role in Civilian Technology Development, on U.S. Strategies for the Children's Vaccine Initiative, on Applications of Biotechnology to Contraceptive Research and Development, and on New Approaches to Breast Cancer Detection and Diagnosis. His research deals with the economics of technological innovation and with the effects of public policies on innovation. He has testified before congressional committees and served as an adviser for the Organisation for Economic Cooperation and Development, various federal agencies, and industrial firms. Dr. Mowery has published numerous academic papers and has written or edited a number of books, including *Ivory Tower and Industrial Innovation: University-Industry Technology Transfer Before and After the Bayh-Dole Act; Paths of Innovation: Technological Change in 20th-Century America; The International Computer Software Industry: A Comparative Study of Industry Evolution and Structure; U.S. Industry in 2000; The Sources of Industrial Leadership; Science and Technology Policy in Interdependent Economies; Technology and the Pursuit of Economic Growth; Technology and Employment: Innovation and Growth in the U.S. Economy; The Impact of Technological Change on Employment and Economic Growth; Technology and the Wealth of Nations;* and *International Collaborative Ventures in U.S. Manufacturing.* His academic awards include the Raymond Vernon Prize from the Association for Public Policy Analysis and Management, the Economic History Association's Fritz Redlich Prize, the *Business History Review*'s Newcomen Prize, and the Cheit Outstanding Teaching Award.

Kathleen M. Rest is executive director of the Union of Concerned Scientists (UCS), where she manages the organization's day-to-day affairs, supervising all program departments on issues ranging from climate change to global security. Dr. Rest is also leading UCS's Climate Solutions Campaign. Dr. Rest came to UCS from the National Institute for Occupational Safety and Health (NIOSH) in the Centers for Disease Control and Prevention, where she was the deputy director for programs. Throughout her tenure at NIOSH, she held several leadership positions, including serving as the Institute's acting director at the time of September 11, 2001, and during the anthrax events that followed. Prior to her work with the federal government, Dr. Rest was an associate professor in the Department of Family and Community Medicine at the University of Massachusetts Medical Center and an adjunct associate professor at the University of Massachusetts School of Public Health. She has extensive experience as a researcher and advisor on occupational and environmental health issues in countries such as the Netherlands, Slovakia, Poland, Romania, Canada, and Greece. Dr. Rest was a founding member of the Association of Occupational and Environmental Clinics, a national nonprofit organization committed to improving the practice of occupational and environmental health through information sharing and collaborative research. She also served as the chairperson of the National Advisory Committee on Occupational Safety and Health. Dr. Rest earned her doctorate in health policy from Boston University and her master's degree in public administration, with a focus on health services, from the University of Arizona.

Thomas A. Saponas was, until his retirement in 2003, the senior vice president and chief technology officer for Agilent Technologies, the $8 billion spin-off of Hewlett Packard Company established in 1999. He had been with Hewlett Packard and Agilent Technologies for 31 years, starting as a research and development engineer. As CTO, Mr. Saponas was responsible for establishing Agilent's long-term technology strategy and directly supervised its central research lab. Prior to this, Mr. Saponas was vice president and general manager of the electronic instruments group at Hewlett Packard (HP), where he led eight divisions and five operations. Earlier, as a general manager, he was also responsible for HP's worldwide research and development, marketing, and manufacturing of oscilloscopes, logic analyzers, and microprocessor development systems. He also had manufacturing responsibility for HP's thin- and thick-film microcircuits. In 1986 Mr. Saponas was selected as a White House Fellow and served 1 year as special assistant to the Secretary of the

Navy. Mr. Saponas has a B.S. degree in computer science and electrical engineering and an M.S. degree in electrical engineering from the University of Colorado.

R. Paul Schaudies is an assistant vice president and division manager of the biological and chemical defense division at Science Applications International Corporation (SAIC). He is a nationally recognized expert in the fields of biological and chemical warfare defense and has served on numerous national level advisory panels for the Defense Intelligence Agency, the Defense Advanced Research Projects Agency, and the Department of Energy. He has 14 years' bench research experience managing laboratories at Walter Reed, at Walter Reed Army Institute of Research, and as a visiting scientist at the National Cancer Institute. He served for 13 years on active duty with the Army Medical Service Corps and separated from service at the rank of lieutenant colonel-select. Dr. Schaudies spent 4 years with the Defense Intelligence Agency as collections manager for biological and chemical defense technologies. As such, he initiated numerous intra-agency collaborations that resulted in accelerated product development in the area of biological warfare agent detection and identification. Dr. Schaudies has served on and chaired numerous technology review and advisory panels for U.S. government agencies. He received his bachelor's degree in chemistry from Wake Forest University and his doctoral degree from Temple University School of Medicine in the department of biochemistry. He has authored 27 scientific manuscripts in the peer-reviewed literature, as well as three book chapters.

Tsung-Tsan Su is the general director of the NanoTechnology Research Center of Taiwan's Industrial Technology Research Institute (ITRI). She also served as the general director of the Office of Planning from August 15, 2000, to December 31, 2004. Before coming to ITRI headquarters, Dr. Su spent 23 years with ITRI's Union Chemical Laboratories, where she held a variety of positions, progressing from her start as a researcher to her final role as deputy general director. She also served for 5 years as the executive director of the National Center for Cleaner Production, Taiwan. Dr. Su holds a B.S. in chemistry from National Tsing-Hua University in Taiwan, a Ph.D. from Princeton University, and a certificate from the international senior management program of Harvard University's Graduate School of Business Administration. She is the recipient of numerous awards from ITRI, including awards for technology contribution, technology promotion and service, and performance, as well as awards for research papers and patents. Dr. Su has also received the Outstanding R&D Program Manager Award of Taiwan's Ministry of Economic Affairs.

Thomas N. Theis is director of physical sciences with the IBM Thomas J. Watson Research Center. He received a B.S. in physics from Rensselaer Polytechnic Institute in 1972 and M.S. and Ph.D. degrees from Brown University in 1974 and 1978, respectively. A portion of his Ph.D. research was done at the Technical University of Munich, where he completed a postdoctoral year before joining IBM Research in 1979. Dr. Theis joined the department of semiconductor science and technology at the IBM Watson Research Center to model the electronic properties of two-dimensional systems. In 1993 he was named senior manager of silicon science and technology, where he was responsible for exploratory materials and process integration work bridging between research and the IBM microelectronics division. He assumed his current position as director of physical sciences in February 1998. Dr. Theis is a member of the Nanotechnology Technical Advisory Group of the President's Council of Advisors on Science and Technology and serves on the National Advisory Board for the National Nanotechnology Infrastructure Network (NNIN). Dr. Theis also serves on the advisory board for the American Institute of Physics Corporate Associates. He is a member of the Physics Policy Committee of the American Physical Society and a member of the Board on Physics and Astronomy of the National Research Council. He is also a member of the IEEE and a fellow of the American Physical Society. He has authored or co-authored over 60 scientific and technical publications.

C

Committee Activities and Participants

WORKSHOP ON MOLECULAR SELF-ASSEMBLY FOR MANUFACTURING
OF MATERIALS AND DEVICES AT THE MOLECULAR SCALE

February 9-11, 2005
Washington, D.C.

Agenda

Session I: Setting the Scene

- E. Clayton Teague, National Nanotechnology Coordination Office/
  National Science and Technology Council
- Celia Merzbacher, National Science and Technology Council/Office of
  Science and Technology Policy

Session II: Establishing a Common Language

- John Randall, Zyvex Corporation
- Ari Requicha, University of Southern California
- Ned Seeman, New York University
- Chris Phoenix, Center for Responsible Nanotechnology

Session III: Setting the Scene

- Scott Mize, Foresight Institute
- Sean Murdock, Nanobusiness Alliance

Overview Presentation

- K. Eric Drexler, Foresight Institute

Session IV: Possibilities and Limitations of Molecular Theory

- Don Eigler, IBM Almaden Research Center
- Peter Cummings, Vanderbilt University
- Ralph Merkle, Georgia Institute of Technology
- K. Eric Drexler, Foresight Institute

Session V: Technology Status and Challenges

- David Forrest, Institute for Molecular Manufacturing
- Carlo Montemagno, University of California, Los Angeles
- Christian Schafmeister, University of Pittsburgh

Session VI: Impacts and Implications

- David Berube, University of South Carolina
- Neil Jacobstein, Institute for Molecular Manufacturing
- David Rejeski, Woodrow Wilson Institute

Participants

Alexander, Catherine, National Nanotechnology Coordination Office
Andrews, Mike, L3 Communications Corporation
Baatar, Chagaan, Office of Naval Research
Bennett, Kristin, Department of Energy
Benney, Tabitha, The National Academies
Berube, David, University of South Carolina
Cardillo, Mark, The Camille and Henry Dreyfus Foundation
Carim, Altaf, Department of Energy
Chang, Julius, Department of Homeland Security
Chen, Hongda, Department of Agriculture
Chernicoff, William, Department of Transportation

Chow, Flora, Environmental Protection Agency
Cummings, Peter, Vanderbilt University
Danello, Mary Ann, Consumer Product Safety Commission
Dastoor, Minoo, National Aeronautics and Space Administration
Dean, Donna, Lewis-Burke Associates LLC
Diamandis, Peter, X PRIZE Foundation
Dillich, Sara, Department of Energy
Drexler, K. Eric, Foresight Institute
Earles, Travis, National Cancer Institute
Eigler, Don, IBM Almaden Research Center
Fezzie, Rachel, Strategic Analysis, Inc.
Fleury, Paul, Yale University
Forrest, David, Naval Surface Warfare Center/Institute for Molecular
    Manufacturing
Glynn, Bridget, Lewis-Burke Associates LLC
Goldstein, Alan, Alfred University
Hartwick, Tom, Snohomish, Washington
Hirschbein, Murray, National Aeronautics and Space Administration
Holliday, Maynard, Evolution Robotics
Irving, Richard, Lakewood Village Community Church
Jacobstein, Neil, Teknowledge Corporation/Institute for Molecular
    Manufacturing
Jhaveri, Sulay, Environmental Protection Agency/American Association for the
    Advancement of Science
Karn, Barbara, Environmental Protection Agency
Keiper, Adam, The New Atlantis
Kozodoy, Peter, Department of State
Levy, Donald, James Franck Institute, University of Chicago
Lippel, Philip, National Nanotechnology Coordination Office
Lipsitt, Harry, Wright State University
Lowe, Terry, Los Alamos National Laboratory
Marlowe, Donald, Food and Drug Administration
Masters, Bettie Sue, University of Texas Health Science Center at San Antonio
Merkle, Ralph, Georgia Institute of Technology, College of Computing
Merzbacher, Celia, National Science and Technology Council/Office of Science
    and Technology Policy
Michelson, Evan, George Washington University
Miller, John, Department of Energy
Miller, Sonia E., Converging Technologies Bar Association
Mize, Scott, Foresight Institute

Montemagno, Carlo, University of California, Los Angeles
Moran, Edward, Deloitte & Touche
Murashov, Vladimir, National Institute for Occupational Safety and Health, Centers for Disease Control and Prevention
Murday, James, Naval Research Laboratory
Murdock, Sean, Nanobusiness Alliance
Murray, Cherry, Lawrence Livermore National Laboratory
Nickelson, Melinda, The National Academies
Phoenix, Chris, Center for Responsible Nanotechnology
Picconatto, Carl, MITRE Corporation
Postek, Michael, National Institute of Standards and Technology
Randall, John, Zyvex Corporation
Rao, Nagesh, U.S. Patent and Trademark Office
Rejeski, David, Woodrow Wilson International Center for Scholars
Requicha, Ari, University of Southern California
Rest, Kathleen, Union of Concerned Scientists
Rothfuss, Christopher, Department of State
Saponas, Tom, Agilent Technologies (retired)
Sayre, Phil, Environmental Protection Agency
Schafmeister, Chris, University of Pittsburgh
Schaudies, Paul, Science Applications International Corporation
Schloss, Jeffrey, National Institutes of Health
Seeman, Ned, New York University
Shull, Robert, National Institute of Standards and Technology
Strine, Linda, Foresight Institute
Su, Tsung-Tsan, Industrial Technology Research Institute (Taiwan)
Teague, Clayton, National Nanotechnology Coordination Office/National Science and Technology Council
Theis, Thomas, Thomas J. Watson Research Center, IBM
Thomas, Treye, Consumer Product Safety Commission
Vorona, Nancy, Virginia's Center for Innovative Technology
Werwa, Eric, Office of Representative Mike Honda, U.S. House of Representatives

BRIEFING TO THE COMMITTEE TO REVIEW
THE NANOTECHNOLOGY INITIATIVE

March 23, 2005
Washington, D.C.

Speakers

- John H. Marburger, III, Office of Science and Technology Policy
- Mihail C. Roco, Subcommittee on Nanoscale Science, Engineering and Technology/National Science Foundation

Charge to NRC Review Committee

- Sharon L. Hays, Office of Science and Technology Policy
- Elizabeth Grossman, Committee on Science, U.S. House of Representatives
- James Wilson, Committee on Science, U.S. House of Representatives
- Jean Toal Eisen, Committee on Commerce, Science and Transportation, U.S. Senate
- Celia Merzbacher, President's Council of Advisors on Science and Technology

NNI Agency Overview and Perspectives

- Patricia Dehmer, Department of Energy
- W. Lance Haworth, National Science Foundation
- David Stepp, Army Research Office, Department of Defense
- Jeffery A. Schloss, National Institutes of Health
- Michael T. Postek, National Institute of Standards and Technology
- Minoo N. Dastoor, National Aeronautics and Space Administration
- Barbara Karn, Environmental Protection Agency
- E. Clayton Teague, National Nanotechnology Coordination Office/ National Science and Technology Council

Participants

Abt, Eileen, The National Academies
Andrews, Mike, L3 Communications Corporation
Auer, Natalie, The Cadmus Group
Bergeson, Lynn, Bergeson & Campbell, LLC

Cardillo, Mark, The Camille and Henry Dreyfus Foundation
Casey, Jeff, Office of Senator Hilary Clinton, U.S. Senate
Dastoor, Minoo, National Aeronautics and Space Administration
Dehmer, Patricia, Department of Energy
DesChamps, Floyd, Senate Committee on Commerce, Science and Transportation
    U.S. Senate
Eisen, Jean Toal, Senate Committee on Commerce, Science and Transportation
    U.S. Senate
Fleury, Paul, Yale University
Frese, Lauren, George Washington University
Germeraad, Paul, Intellectual Assets, Inc.
Goldstein, Alan, Alfred University
Good, Mary, University of Arkansas at Little Rock
Grossman, Elizabeth, Committee on Science, U.S. House of Representatives
Gustafson, Carl, The National Academies
Hartwick, Tom, Snohomish, Washington
Haworth, W. Lance, National Science Foundation
Hays, Sharon, Office of Science and Technology Policy, Executive Office of the
    President
Helble, Joe, Office of Sen. Joseph Lieberman, U.S. Senate
Hirschbein, Murray, National Aeronautics and Space Administration
Holliday, Maynard, Evolution Robotics
Karn, Barbara, Environmental Protection Agency
Levy, Donald, James Franck Institute, University of Chicago
Livingston, Richard, Federal Highway Administration
Lowe, Terry, Los Alamos National Laboratory
Marburger, John H., III, Office of Science and Technology Policy, Executive
    Office of the President
Masters, Bettie Sue, University of Texas Health Science Center at San Antonio
Mehan, G. Tracy, III, The Cadmus Group
Meierhoefer, Melissa, Georgia Tech Office of Federal Relations
Merzbacher, Celia, National Science and Technology Council/Office of Science
    and Technology Policy
Miller, Sonia E., Converging Technologies Bar Association
Moran, Edward, Deloitte & Touche
Murray, Cherry, Lawrence Livermore National Laboratory
Postek, Michael, National Institute of Standards and Technology
Rest, Kathleen, Union of Concerned Scientists
Roco, Mihail, National Science Foundation
Rothfuss, Christopher, Department of State

Saponas, Tom, Agilent Technologies (retired)
Schadler, Harvey, GE Corporate Research and Development (retired)
Schaudies, Paul, Science Applications International Corporation
Schloss, Jeff, National Institutes of Health
Stepp, David, Department of Defense, Army Research Office
Su, Tsung-Tsan, Industrial Technology Research Institute (Taiwan)
Teague, Clayton, National Nanotechnology Coordination Office/National Science and Technology Council
Tinkle, Sally, National Institute of Environmental Health Sciences
Williams, James, Ohio State University
Wilson, James, House Committee on Science, U.S. House of Representatives

WORKSHOP ON RESPONSIBLE DEVELOPMENT OF NANOTECHNOLOGY

March 24-25, 2005
Washington, D.C.

Agenda

Session 1: Societal Dimensions of Nanotechnology

- Clayton Teague, National Nanotechnology Coordination Office/National Science and Technology Council
- Frances Schrotter, American National Standards Institute
- Barbara Karn, Environmental Protection Agency
- Vicki Colvin, Rice University/American National Standards Institute—Nanotechnology Standards Panel
- Daniel Gamota, Motorola, Inc./Institute of Electrical and Electronics Engineers

Session 2: Biomedical and Environmental Applications and Implications

- Andrew Maynard, National Institute for Occupational Safety and Health
- Sally Tinkle, National Institute of Environmental Health Sciences
- Vicki Colvin, Rice University/American National Standards Institute—Nanotechnology Standards Panel
- David Warheit, DuPont

Lunch Dialogue (Teleconference) with the Royal Society (UK)

- Ann Dowling, University of Cambridge
- Rachel Quinn, The Royal Society
- Mark E. Welland, University of Cambridge

Session 3: Establishing Standards and Guidelines for Responsible Economic Development

- Jack Solomon, Praxair, Inc.
- Carol Henry, American Chemistry Council
- Lori Perine, American Forest and Paper Association
- Pat Picariello, ASTM International
- Stephen Harper, Intel Corporation

Session 4: Defensive Technologies, Human Enhancement, and Ethical Issues

- William Peters, Institute for Soldier Nanotechnologies, Massachusetts Institute of Technology
- Debra Rolison, Naval Research Laboratory
- George Khushf, Center for Bioethics, University of South Carolina
- Rosalyn Berne, Nanotechnology Ethics, University of Virginia

Session 5: Societal Dimensions, Public Awareness, Education, and Workforce Training

- Jane Macoubrie, North Carolina State University
- Kristen Kulinowski, Rice University
- Richard Denison, Environmental Defense
- Dietram A. Scheufele, University of Wisconsin, Madison

Participants

Abt, Eileen, The National Academies
Ali, Mohammed, Nanophase Technologies Corporation
Alwood, Jim, Environmental Protection Agency
Andrews, Mike, L3 Communications Corporation
Auer, Natalie, The Cadmus Group
Bahadori, Tina, American Chemistry Council
Bawa, Raj, Bawa Biotechnology Consulting, LLC
Berne, Rosalyn, University of Virginia
Cardillo, Mark, The Camille and Henry Dreyfus Foundation
Chow, Flora, Environmental Protection Agency
Colvin, Vicki, Rice University
Dastoor, Minoo, National Aeronautics and Space Administration
Denison, Richard, Environmental Defense
Diamandis, Peter, X PRIZE Foundation
Dowling, Ann P., University of Cambridge (via teleconference)
Fezzie, Rachel, Strategic Analysis, Inc.
Gamota, Daniel, Motorola, Inc./Institute of Electrical and Electronics Engineers
Germeraad, Paul, Intellectual Assets, Inc.
Gilman, Paul, Oak Ridge Center for Advanced Studies
Goldstein, Alan, Alfred University
Good, Mary, University of Arkansas at Little Rock
Graham, Judith, American Chemistry Council
Gustafson, Carl, The National Academies

Harper, Steve, Intel Corporation
Hartwick, Tom, Snohomish, Washington
Helble, Joe, Office of Senator Joseph Lieberman, U.S. Senate
Henry, Carol, American Chemistry Council
Hirschbein, Murray, National Aeronautics and Space Administration
Holliday, Maynard, Evolution Robotics
Hurd, Jim, NanoScience Exchange
Ikukawa, Hiroshi, Embassy of Japan
Jordan, Willam, Environmental Protection Agency
Karn, Barbara, Environmental Protection Agency
Khushf, George, University of South Carolina
Kozodoy, Peter, Department of State
Kulinowski, Kristen, Rice University
Lerman, Daniel, National Institutes of Health
Levy, Donald, James Franck Institute, University of Chicago
Lippel, Philip H., National Nanotechnology Coordination Office
Lowe, Terry, Los Alamos National Laboratory
Macoubrie, Jane, North Carolina State University
Marin, Mark, Lewis-Burke Associates LLC
Masters, Bettie Sue, University of Texas Health Science Center at San Antonio
Maynard, Andrew, National Institute for Occupational Safety and Health,
    Centers for Disease Control and Prevention
Mazza, Carl, Environmental Protection Agency
Mehan, G. Tracy III, The Cadmus Group
Merzbacher, Celia, National Science and Technology Council/Office of Science
    and Technology Policy
Michelson, Evan, George Washington University
Miller, Sonia E., Converging Technologies Bar Association
Mize, Scott, Foresight Institute
Moore, Julia, National Science Foundation
Moran, Edward, Deloitte & Touche
Morris, Jeff, Environmental Protection Agency
Murashov, Vladimir, National Institute for Occupational Safety and Health,
    Centers for Disease Control and Prevention
Murray, Cherry, Lawrence Livermore National Laboratory
Needham, Cynthia, ICAN Productions, Ltd.
Perine, Lori, American Forest and Paper Association
Peters, William, Institute of Solder Nanotechnologies, Massachusetts Institute of
    Technology
Peterson, Christine, Foresight Institute

Phipps, Pat, Daily Environment Report, BNA, Inc.

Picariello, Pat, ASTM-International

Picconatto, Carl, MITRE Corporation

Quinn, Rachel, The Royal Society (via teleconference)

Rest, Kathleen, Union of Concerned Scientists

Roberson, Scott, Strategic Analysis, Inc.

Roco, Mihail, National Science Foundation

Rolison, Debra, Naval Research Laboratory

Rothfuss, Christopher, Department of State

Saponas, Tom, Agilent Technologies (retired)

Savage, Nora, Environmental Protection Agency

Sayre, Philip, Environmental Protection Agency

Schadler, Harvey, GE Corporate Research and Development (Retired)

Schaffer, Keri, Environmental Protection Agency

Schaudies, Paul, Science Applications International Corporation

Scheufele, Dietram, University of Wisconsin, Madison

Schloss, Jeff, National Institutes of Health

Schrotter, Frances, American National Standards Institute

Shindo, Hideo, NEDO (Japan)

Smith, Richard, Foresight Institute/Nanoverse LLC

Solomon, Jack, Praxair, Inc.

Street, Anita, Environmental Protection Agency

Su, Tsung-Tsan, Industrial Technology Research Institute (Taiwan)

Teague, Clayton, National Nanotechnology Coordination Office/National Science and Technology Council

Theis, Thomas, Thomas J. Watson Research Center, IBM

Thomas, Treye A., Consumer Product Safety Commission

Tinkle, Sally, National Institute of Environmental Health Sciences

Utterback, Dennis, Environmental Protection Agency

Valle, Eduardo, The National Academies

Warheit, David, DuPont

Welland, Mark, University of Cambridge (via teleconference)

Williams, James, Ohio State University

Wind, Marilyn, Consumer Product Safety Commission

Wrightson, Patricia, The National Academies

PRESENTATIONS ON TECHNOLOGY TRANSFER
AND ECONOMIC IMPACTS

June 27-28, 2005
Washington, D.C.

Agenda

Session 1: The State of the NNI

- Floyd Kvamme, President's Council of Advisors on Science and Technology
- E. Clayton Teague, National Nanotechnology Coordination Office/ National Science and Technology Council
- Mihail C. Roco, Subcommittee on Nanoscale Science, Engineering and Technology/National Science Foundation

Session 2: The Unique Nature of Nanotech

- Marlene Bourne, EmTech Research
- Derrick Boston, Guth|Christopher LLP
- Bart F. Romanowicz, Nano Science and Technology Institute

Session 3: The Unique Impacts of Nanotech on the Economy

- Matthew Nordan, Lux Research, Inc.
- Andrew Dunn, Cientifica Ltd.
- JoAnne Feeney, Punk, Ziegel & Company

Session 4: The Impact of NNI Funding on Industrial Base Development

- Thomas A. Kalil, University of California, Berkeley/Center for American Progress
- Sean Murdock, NanoBusiness Alliance

Session 5: The State of Technology Transition to Achieve Government Agency Missions

- Minoo Dastoor, National Aeronautics and Space Administration
- Barbara Karn, Environmental Protection Agency
- David Stepp, Army Research Office, Department of Defense

Participants

Albert, Josh, Office of Senator Hilary Clinton, U.S. Senate
Alexander, Catherine B., National Nanotechnology Coordination Office
Andrews, Mike, L3 Communications Corporation
Anquetil, Patrick, Susquehanna Financial Group
Berube, David, NanoCenter, University of South Carolina
Boston, Derrick, Guth|Christopher LLP
Bourne, Marlene, EmTech Research/Small Times
Burgin, Deborah, Environmental Protection Agency
Burns, Marshall, X PRIZE Foundation
Cardillo, Mark, The Camille and Henry Dreyfus Foundation
Carim, Altaf H., Department of Energy
Chow, Flora, Environmental Protection Agency
Cunanan, Crystal, ReVision Optics
Dastoor, Minoo, National Aeronautics and Space Administration
Downing, Greg, National Cancer Institute
Dunn, Andrew, Cientifica
Earles, Travis, National Cancer Institute
Feeney, JoAnne, Punk, Ziegel & Company
Germeraad, Paul, Intellectual Assets, Inc.
Goldstein, Alan, Alfred University
Good, Mary, University Arkansas at Little Rock
Grodzinski, Piotr, National Cancer Institute
Hartwick, Tom, Snohomish, Washington
Helble, Joe, Office of Sen. Joseph Lieberman, U.S. Senate
Henkin, Josh, Office of the Secretary of Defense, Department of Defense
Holdridge, Geoff, National Nanotechnology Coordination Office
Irving, Richard, Lakewood Village Community Church
Jacobson, Ken, Manufacturing and Technology News
Kalil, Thomas A., Center for American Progress, University of California
Karn, Barbara, Environmental Protection Agency
Kousvelari, Eleni, National Institute of Dental and Craniofacial Research,
    National Institutes of Health
Kovacs, Andrew, Committee on Science, U.S. House of Representatives
Kozodoy, Peter, Department of State
Kvamme, Floyd, Kleiner Perkins Caulfield & Byer
Levy, Donald, James Franck Institute, University of Chicago
Lewinski, Nastassja, Rice University
Lingle, Stephen, Environmental Protection Agency

Lippel, Philip H., National Nanotechnology Coordination Office
Lipsitt, Harry, Wright State University
Lowe, Terry, Los Alamos National Laboratory
Merrill, Steve, the National Academies
Merzbacher, Celia, National Science and Technology Council/Office of Science and Technology Policy
Miller, Sonia E., Converging Technologies Bar Association
Moran, Edward, Deloitte & Touche
Morrissey, Susan, Chemical & Engineering News, American Chemical Society
Mowery, David, University of California, Berkeley
Murashov, Vladimir, National Institute for Occupational Safety and Health, Centers for Disease Control and Prevention
Murray, Cherry, Lawrence Livermore National Laboratory
Noble, Eric U., Department of State
Nordan, Matthew, Lux Research, Inc.
Postek, Michael, National Institute of Standards and Technology
Rao, Nagesh, U.S. Patent and Trademark Office
Rejeski, David, Woodrow Wilson International Center for Scholars
Roco, Michael, National Science Foundation
Romanowicz, Bart, Nano Science and Technology Institute
Schadler, Harvey, GE Corporate Research and Development (retired)
Schaudies, Paul, Science Applications International Corporation
Schloss, Jeffery, National Human Genome Research Institute, National Institutes of Health
Shull, Robert, National Institute of Standards and Technology
Slavick, Jennifer, Environmental Protection Agency
Stepp, David, Army Research Office, Department of Defense
Su, Tsung-Tsan, Industrial Technology Research Institute (Taiwan)
Teague, Clayton, National Nanotechnology Coordination Office/National Science and Technology Council
Tinkle, Sally, National Institute of Environmental Health Sciences
Walker, Ken, Luna nanoWorks
Williams, James, Ohio State University

WORKSHOP ON PROGRAM MANAGEMENT
AND SCIENTIFIC ACCOMPLISHMENTS

August 25-26, 2005
Washington, D.C.

Agenda

Session 1: Program Management of the NNI

- Clayton Teague, National Nanotechnology Coordination Office/National Science and Technology Council
- Kristin Bennett, Department of Energy
- Norris Alderson, Food and Drug Administration
- Jeffery Schloss, Human Genome Research Institute, National Institutes of Health
- Irene Brahmakulam, Office of Management and Budget
- Celia Merzbacher, President's Council on Science and Technology
- James Murday, Naval Research Laboratory
- Michael T. Postek, National Institute of Standards and Technology
- Mihail C. Roco, Subcommittee on Nanoscale Science, Engineering and Technology/National Science Foundation
- Treye Thomas, Consumer Product Safety Commission

Dinner Speaker

- Kent Hughes, Woodrow Wilson International Center for Scholars

Session 2: Scientific Impact of NNI

- Matthew Tirrell, University of California, Santa Barbara
- Samuel Stupp, Northwestern University
- Moungi Bawendi, Massachusetts Institute of Technology
- Ellen Williams, University of Maryland
- Lou Brus, Columbia University

Session 3: Nanopatents and Intellectual Property

- Stephen Maebius, Foley & Lardner LLP
- Bruce Kisliuk, U.S. Patent and Trademark Office

Participants

Alderson, Norris, Food and Drug Administration

Andrews, Mike, L3 Communications Corporation

Bawendi, Moungi, Massachusetts Institute of Technology

Bennett, Kristin, Department of Energy

Brahmakulam, Irene, Office of Management and Budget

Brus, Louis, Columbia University

Cardillo, Mark, The Camille and Henry Dreyfus Foundation

Chow, Flora, Environmental Protection Agency

Cunanan, Crystal, ReVision Optics

Dastoor, Minoo, National Aeronautics and Space Administration

Fleury, Paul, Yale University

Germeraad, Paul, Intellectual Assets, Inc.

Goldstein, Alan, Alfred University

Good, Mary, University of Arkansas at Little Rock

Gross, Mihal, Office of Naval Research

Haworth, W. Lance, National Science Foundation

Henkin, Josh, Department of Defense

Hirschbein, Murray, National Aeronautics and Space Administration

Holdridge, Geoff, National Nanotechnology Coordination Office

Holliday, Maynard, Evolution Robotics

Hughes, Kent, Woodrow Wilson International Center for Scholars

Jhaveri, Sulay, Environmental Protection Agency/American Association for the Advancement of Science

Karn, Barbara, Environmental Protection Agency

Kisliuk, Bruce, U.S. Patent and Trademark Office

Levy, Donald, James Franck Institute, University of Chicago

Lippel, Philip H., National Nanotechnology Coordination Office

Lipsitt, Harry, Wright State University

Lowe, Terry, Los Alamos National Laboratory

MacDonald, Neil, Federal Technology Watch

Maebius, Stephen, Foley & Lardner, LLP

Masters, Bettie Sue, University of Texas Health Science Center at San Antonio

Merzbacher, Celia, President's Council of Advisors on Science and Technology

Michelson, Evan, George Washington University

Miller, Sonia E., Converging Technologies Bar Association

Moran, Edward, Deloitte & Touche

Mowery, David, University of California, Berkeley

Murashov, Vladimir, National Institute for Occupational Safety and Health,
    Centers for Disease Control and Prevention
Murday, James, Naval Research Laboratory
Murray, Cherry, Lawrence Livermore National Laboratory (via teleconference)
Postek, Michael, National Institute of Standards and Technology
Rejeski, David, Woodrow Wilson International Center for Scholars
Rest, Kathy, Union of Concerned Scientists
Roco, Mihail, Subcommittee on Nanoscale Science, Engineering and Technology/
    National Science Foundation
Samulski, Ed, Department of State/University of North Carolina at Chapel Hill
Schaudies, Paul, Science Applications International Corporation
Schloss, Jeffery, Human Genome Research Institute, National Institutes of Health
Stepp, David, Department of Defense, Army Research Office
Stupp, Sam, Northwestern University
Teague, Clayton, National Nanotechnology Coordination Office/National Science
    and Technology Council
Theis, Thomas, Thomas J. Watson Research Center, IBM
Thomas, Treye, Consumer Product Safety Commission
Tirrell, Matthew, University of California, Santa Barbara (via videoconference)
Turner, Victor, National Nanotechnology Coordination Office
Wang, Yan, Science and Technology Office, Embassy of China
Williams, Ellen, University of Maryland
Williams, James, Ohio State University

INDIVIDUALS INTERVIEWED AND THEIR CORPORATE AFFILIATIONS

Larry Bock, CEO, Nanosys, Palo Alto, California

Uma Chowdhry, Vice President of Central R&D, DuPont, Wilmington, Delaware

Daniel Gamota, Distinguished Member of the Technical Staff and Senior Manager of the Printed Electronics Solutions Department, Motorola, Schaumburg, Illinois

Paolo Gargini, Director of Technology Strategy, Intel Corporation, Santa Clara, California

Magnus Gittins, President and Chief Executive Officer, Advance Nanotech, New York, New York

Michael Helmus, Senior Vice President, BioPharma, Advance Nanotech, Inc., New York, New York

Michael Idelchik, Director, GE Global Research, Niskayuna, New York

Amit Kumar, President and CEO, CombiMatrix Corporation, Mukilteo, Washington

David Macdonald, President and CEO, Nanomix, Emeryville, California

Hash Pakbaz, Vice President, Business Development, Cambrios Technologies Corp., Mountain View, California

Sharon Smith, Director, Advanced Technology, Lockheed Martin Corporation, Bethesda, Maryland

D

Workshop Proceedings: Responsible Development of Nanotechnology

The Workshop on Responsible Development of Nanotechnology was held on March 24-25, 2005, in Washington, D.C., as part of this study to discuss the need for standards, guidelines, and strategies for ensuring the responsible development of nanotechnology. The presentations included information on NNI programs and the status of standards and guidelines for nanotechnology R&D, and some also identified areas in need of further planning and action.

SESSION I:
SOCIETAL DIMENSIONS OF NANOTECHNOLOGY

E. Clayton Teague
Director,
National Nanotechnology Coordination Office

The National Nanotechnology Initiative (NNI) has focused on the societal dimensions of nanotechnology since its inception. Even during the planning stages, federal investments were balanced to foster innovation in nanoscale science and technology while addressing environmental, health, and safety (EHS) implications. Other areas of interest include education-related activities, such as development of materials for schools, undergraduate programs, technical training, and public outreach; and broad societal implications of nanotechnology, including economic, workforce, ethical, and legal implications. The NNI has continued to make EHS issues important by establishing societal dimensions as one of seven program component areas (PCAs).

The unique properties of nanoscale materials make focusing on the societal implications critical. For example, the characteristics of new nanostructures require full analysis and investigation. The chemical and physical properties of nanoscale gold clusters differ greatly from those of more macroscopic metallic forms. Materials at such dimensions show unusual quantum effects that can dominate surface and electronic properties. However, the unique properties of these materials are a double-edged sword: they can be tailored for beneficial properties but also have unknown consequences, such as new toxicological and environmental effects. NNI's strategic plan identifies the importance of societal dimensions of nanotechnologies, and also focuses on responsible development of nanomanufacturing and safety. In 2004, memos from the Office of Management and Budget (OMB) and the Office of Science and Technology Policy (OSTP) to federal agency heads reiterated this focus. Those memos noted that "agencies should support research on the various societal implications of the nascent technology" by placing "a high priority on research on human health and environmental issues . . . [and] cross-agency approaches."

The result is that 11 federal agencies have allocated $38.5 million to R&D focused on the EHS implications of nanotechnology, and $42.6 million to R&D on ethical and legal issues and public communication. These funds represent 8 percent of all federal funds devoted to nanoscale materials and devices.

NNI is directly pursuing EHS initiatives on several fronts. First, NNI is encouraging agencies to develop data on the potential toxicity of nanomaterials. For example, in October 2003, the National Toxicology Program under the Department of Health and Human Services began to study the potential toxicological effects of titanium dioxide nanoparticles, single-walled carbon nanotubes, and quantum dots. NNI is further devoting $1 million to research on the toxicity of nanomaterials at such institutions as the University of Houston and the University of Rochester. The National Cancer Institute's Nanotechnology Characterization Laboratory has developed a characterization cascade for use in preclinical evaluations of nanomaterials intended for cancer therapeutics. The Environmental Protection Agency (EPA), National Science Foundation (NSF), and National Institute for Occupational Safety and Health (NIOSH) will fund research from a competitive solicitation that addresses potentially harmful aspects of nanomaterials, whether nanomaterials bioaccumulate, and whether they pose health and environmental risks. This research will also focus on the fate, transport, and transformation of nanoscale materials after they enter the body and the environment.

In 2004, NIOSH established the Nanotechnology Research Center (NTRC) to coordinate nanotechnology research across the Institute. NTRC's mission is "to provide national and world leadership for research into the application of nanoparticles and nanomaterials in occupational safety and health and the implications of nanoparticles and nanomaterials for work-related injury and illness." In 2005, NIOSH published a Strategic Plan for nanotechnology research. The goals are to prevent work-related injuries and illnesses caused by nanoparticles and nanomaterials; apply nanotechnology products to prevent such injuries and illnesses; promote healthy workplaces through intervention, recommendations, and capacity building; and enhance global workplace safety through national and international collaborations.

In August 2003, NNI formed the Nanotechnology Environmental and Health Implications (NEHI) Working Group to coordinate federal programs and efforts among research and regulatory agencies. This group, which meets regularly, is fostering standards for nanotechnology and advancing the understanding of environmental implications and the impact on workers' health. The group is also documenting practices recommended by NIOSH and the Occupational Safety and Health Administration for working with such materials. NNI is further identifying specific R&D needed to improve regulatory decision making on nanotechnology, and helping regulatory agencies develop websites and position statements on the responsible use of these technologies. NNI also formed a Nanotechnology Public Engagement Group to develop approaches for communicating more effectively with the public.

NNI is also trying to promote multidisciplinary education related to nanoscale science and engineering, and to ensure that the nation's labor force has the skills and knowledge to work with nanotechnology. NNI has also worked to ensure that all stakeholders can participate in public debate and decision making regarding nanotechnology. Toward this end, NNI not only maintains its own website but has also created websites and outreach activities at federally funded nanotechnology centers and Department of Energy user facilities.

NSF's Nanoscale Informal Science Education Network was announced in October 2005. This award will support a national network of science museums, providing informal educational activities for schoolchildren as well as adults. NSF funding is also creating two Centers for Nanotechnology in Society, one at Arizona Statue University, and the other at University of California at Santa Barbara. Through a network of social scientists, economists, and nanotechnology researchers, each Center will address key issues regarding the societal implications of nanoscience and nanotechnology. The Centers will also formulate a long-term vision for addressing EHS concerns; collaborate with partners or affiliates on the responsible use of nanotechnology; involve a wide range of stakeholders; develop a clearinghouse for information on communicating about nanoscience and nanotechnology, and engage the public in meaningful dialogue.

NSF has further funded a Center for Learning and Teaching in Nanoscale Science and Engineering, which focuses on grades 7-12 and the undergraduate level. The Department of Defense (DOD) collaborates with NSF in the NSF-Navy Civilian Service Fellowship/Scholarship program. This program seeks students at the bachelors, masters, or doctoral level in science, technology, engineering, and mathematics who wish to commit a portion of their careers to serve at a Navy R&D center. The NCI Alliance for Nanotechnology in Cancer is supporting the education, training, and career development of postdoctoral as well as mid-career investigators for multidisciplinary nano-oncology research.

NNI intends to perform R&D on environment, health, and safety in parallel with the discovery of new nanoscale materials and properties. NNI funding of EHS and societal issues has therefore grown substantially along with its investments in nanotechnology. Regulatory mechanisms for assessing and regulating environmental impact, workplace safety, and other health risks are being mobilized. Research at federal laboratories and in private industry and academia will help determine how nanotechnology-based materials may differ from conventional ones in their implications for public health and the environment.

Vicki Colvin
Center for Biological and Environmental Nanotechnology
Rice University

As an NSF center of excellence on nanotechnology, the Center for Biological and Environmental Nanotechnology has focused on the challenge of communicating the risks of nanotechnology to the public. Interactions with the public have made the center keenly aware of the importance of standards and terminology in defining this emerging technology and developing it responsibly. For example, when it is burned, diesel fuel emits carbon ultrafine particles that are dangerous to human health. However, the properties of such particles differ from those of engineered nanomaterials, such as fullerenes and carbon nanotubes. Yet discussions with journalists have indicated that the distinctions were not initially clear to the public and required further attention from researchers to define nanomaterials precisely.

Classifying nanoscale particles and identifying relevant characteristics and properties are important steps in preventing generalizations about all matter at the nanoscale. Without distinct classifications, the public too often places all nanoscale particles and nanotechnologies under one giant umbrella. For example, researchers have accumulated data on the toxicology of waste particles such as those that result from burning diesel. However, nanoparticles manufactured for a specific use may not carry the same risks. Without more accurate nomenclature, the public has no way of differentiating the impacts of incidental versus engineered materials.

Questions about nomenclature and standards affect the regulatory process directly. For example, buyers of carbon 60 now receive a Material Safety Data Sheet that labels elemental carbon and carbon black as "nuisance dust"—even though carbon 60 differs from those two substances. Like names for polymers, nomenclature for nanomaterials should indicate their surface type, as that information can shed light on how they interact with their environment.

Although industry consortia usually drive efforts to create products, nomenclature, and standards, the business case for a single investment in nanotechnology products is not yet compelling outside the electronics industry. Nanotechnology is still embryonic, and most companies don't see where standards fit into their bottom line. A large fraction of participants in the development of terminology and standards will therefore come from academia.

The top level of terminology—that is, how best to divide nanomaterials between physics and chemistry—is the most controversial, so the need for multidisciplinary coordination in determining nomenclature is great. Although ANSI will coordinate and adjudicate this activity, the American Society for Testing and Materials (ASTM) International has established the Committee E56 on Nanotechnology to actually create the standards for nanotechnology. ASTM has recruited researchers to write the documentation that informs the voluntary process for developing consensus on these standards. Subgroups have formed to author documentation on terminology and nomenclature, metrology, and EHS issues.

Barbara Karn
U.S. Environmental Protection Agency

NNI's definition of nanotechnology has three aspects. First, it deals with materials with at least one dimension between 1 and 100 nm. Next, it includes materials whose properties change because of their size. Finally, nanotechnology involves the ability to create unique structures with fundamentally new building blocks of atomic and molecular clusters. The ultimate goal is the ability to assemble essentially anything from scratch.

Discussion of responsible development of nanotechnology is complex because it includes more than a single material or even class of materials, encompassing instead materials with a wide range of properties and products with many uses. Nanotechnology also encompasses a wide range of different industrial sectors, including but not limited to the automotive and chemical industries, pharmacology, medicine, communications, electronics, and information technologies. Consumer products, equipment for manufacturing nanomaterials and products, and advanced instrumentation are already on the market. Nanotechnology is also converging with other technologies, such as biotechnology and information technology, to form even more powerful new scientific and industrial approaches.

First-generation nanoparticles—which include, for example, polymer fillers, ceramic particles, and nanoclays—are "passive," in that they have a single function and are usually incorporated into other materials. Second-generation nanotechnologies are more active, smart, and multifunctional structures. The third generation—nanosystems, and, finally, systems of nanosystems—will appear over the next 5 to 10 years. These more advanced nanomaterials and products will include various assembly techniques, nanoscale architectures and networking, biomimetic materials, therapeutics, and targeted drug delivery.

Regulators of these technologies can take two approaches in protecting human health and the environment, based on their view of nanotechnology. One school of thought views nanotechnology as an inherently continuous extension of existing fields. If that is the case, the current regulatory system can keep up with development and adequately address the potential impacts of this new technology. Another school of thought believes that nanotechnology will prove revolutionary scientifically, industrially, and socially. In the latter case, regulators need to develop more nimble approaches to address these paradigm shifts. Which viewpoint is chosen will determine how regulators approach responsible research and development of nanotechnology.

NNI bears some obligation to ensure responsible development of nanotechnology because it oversees $1.2 billion in federal funding—2 to 3 percent of which is devoted to research on environmental, health, and safety implications. Industry is also a key source for researching the potential impacts of nanotechnology, as the field may account for a $1 trillion piece of the nation's economic pie in 5 to 10 years.

Reflecting growing international dialog on responsible R&D on nanotechnology, many countries are focusing on both applications and implications for the environment and human health. as well as its socioeconomic and ethical implications. As evidence of this concern, the Organisation for Economic Co-operation and Development proposed a special session on the impact of nanotechnology on chemical safety at the June 2005 meeting of the Chemicals Committee and the Working Party on Chemicals, Pesticides, and Biotechnology.

For its part, the U.S. Environmental Protection Agency is investigating potential applications and implications of nanotechnology. The former includes sensing pollution, remediating hazardous waste, ensuring green manufacturing, and producing green energy. The latter includes life cycle assessment, toxicology, exposure, bioavailability, fate and transport in the environment, and bioaccumulation of nanomaterials.

Green nanotechnology offers the opportunity to manufacture materials atom by atom to produce less waste and pollution, to create lightweight, stronger products that use less energy and fewer materials in their manufacture, and to ensure better industrial controls to minimize pollution. Two examples include synthesizing nanotubes using microwaves to reduce energy use in their manufacture, and the use of molecular nanolithography for bottom-up assembly of nanoscale electronic devices. Nanotechnology also offers the opportunity to clean up hazardous waste. An example is remediating groundwater contaminated with trichloroethylene by using iron nanoparticles, which more easily move through the soil and are more reactive than larger particles due to their increased surface area.

EPA's nanotechnology research program embraces six thrusts. These include building a community of researchers that work in both nanotechnology and the environment, institutionalizing nanotechnology within EPA's mission, ensuring consideration of EHS concerns in other federally funded research programs, working with industry to ensure that it develops nanotechnology responsibly, providing international leadership in EHS, and providing education and outreach to the public. Overall, EPA sees itself as the conscience of NNI to make sure that EHS issues are considered in all NNI agencies' research.

Research on nanotechnology has made huge strides within the past year. Nanoscale products have become a reality, nano-related green manufacturing is accelerating, and the research in toxicology of nanotechnology has become a familiar concept. Myriad professional societies are addressing EHS-related issues, and NNI's EHS activities continue to grow. EPA sees its central goal as using nanotechnology to clean up existing environmental damage and prevent future damage, to ensure a sustainable future.

Daniel Gamota
Motorola and the Institute of Electrical and Electronics Engineers

The now infamous McKinsey report predicted that by 2000 only a million cell phones would be in use. That prediction vastly underestimated the market, because it did not recognize that today's cell phones would contain as much horsepower as humanity used to go to the Moon in 1969. Silicon's intrinsic properties have not changed. Rather, nanoscale features now enable cell phones to work faster at a given cost, and provide higher performance within the same physical dimensions and weight.

Given the revolutionary nature of nanotechnology, the Institute of Electrical and Electronics Engineers (IEEE) resolved to spearhead work on standards for characterizing the new technology, which could propel hundreds of electronics and photonics products. Specifically, IEEE has partnered with other standards-

developing organizations to develop certificates of compliance and standard operating procedures for high-volume manufacturing, to ensure reliable output, to
protect workers, and to address environmental concerns.

IEEE first convened a workshop for representatives from industry, academia,
and international laboratories to examine the kinds of standards needed for
nanoscale materials, devices, and systems. IEEE then established a working group
to draft standard methods for measuring the electrical properties of carbon nanotubes. The result is consensus-based standards—posted on the Web and circu-
lated via the Internet—on how to electronically characterize carbon nanotubes.
Because characterizing nanomaterials requires cross-disciplinary expertise, IEEE
also worked with Semiconductor Materials and Equipment International (SEMI)
and ASTM International to propose standards for the types and characteristics of
nanoparticles, and nomenclature and terminology for nanotechnology.

Without such standards, researchers cannot duplicate experiments performed
by others and confirm their results. Standards will ensure a seamless interface
between silicon-based devices and nanoelectronics to provide interoperability
between mature and revolutionary technologies. Interoperability standards enabled
the creation and growth of industries such as Web services, storage networks, and
cell phones. Standards are critical to enable industry to purchase well-characterized
nanoparticles from different suppliers—start-up companies are already selling
carbon nanotubes—and design early nanotechnology-based products that will
likely interface with existing technologies.

SESSION II
BIOMEDICAL AND ENVIRONMENTAL APPLICATIONS
AND IMPLICATIONS

Andrew Maynard[1]
Senior Service Fellow, National Institute for Occupational Safety and Health

The responsible use of nanotechnology raises two key questions. Do the unique
features of engineered nanomaterials lead to unique safety and health risks? How
can we maximize the benefits of nanotechnology while minimizing the risks from
unintended consequences?

Information on what exactly is different about these materials, and the signifi-
cance of their structure, will prove key to answering these questions. Important
structural elements that can affect the chemical and biological features of these

---

[1]Currently a senior advisor to the Project on Emerging Nanotechnologies at the Woodrow Wilson
International Center for Scholars.

materials include their size, shape, surface area, and surface activity. In addition, physical properties, such as surface charge density and optical and magnetic phenomena, may be of importance.

Engineered nanomaterials, which potentially present new challenges for human health, have two attributes: they can enter the body, and their nanostructure can lead to specific biological activity. Such materials can include nanoparticles that can be inhaled or absorbed through the skin, such as aerosols, powders, suspensions, and slurries, as well as materials that degrade during grinding, cutting, machining, or other occupational use. To address these risks responsibly, we need to understand several critical issues, including exposure routes, doses, and toxicity. Standard risk analysis requires characterizing these materials and exposures accurately, as well as conveying the resulting information to people who need it.

We are not starting with a blank slate in answering these questions. The field of occupational hygiene has matured considerably, and analysts have accumulated extensive information about how people respond to hazardous materials. We can extrapolate from such information—such as how a material's surface area and activity influence the biological response to it—to investigate nanotechnology. For example, information on the inhalation hazard of insoluble aerosols with different surface chemistries can contribute to assessing new nanomaterials. Although nanotechnology may be revolutionary as well as evolutionary, we do have a starting point in dealing with risks.

The National Institute for Occupational Safety and Health (NIOSH) is congressionally mandated to take the lead in investigating risks related to occupational safety and health. NIOSH has already focused significantly on three aspects of exposure to nanoparticles: what kind of research on risk is needed, which partnerships are essential to investigating such risks, and how best to communicate the resulting information. For example, the agency is tapping internationally recognized experts to characterize toxicity, exposures, and the impacts on human health of single-walled carbon nanotubes. The agency convened the first two international meetings on nanotechnology and occupational health to jump-start a global initiative drawing together people from different sectors to address these issues. NIOSH is also developing a website to broadcast information on nanotechnology and occupational health, including not only the toxicity and risk of engineered nanomaterials but also effective practices for working with them.

Occupational safety and health are key societal issues that require attention for the responsible development of nanotechnology. If workers are exposed to unconventional nanostructures on the job, we must address their impact to ensure safe workplaces. Existing knowledge provides a starting point for addressing these risks, and we can rely on evolutionary approaches in evaluating the health impacts of "simple nanomaterials." However, nanotechnology challenges conventional approaches, and we need to address the potential consequences and impacts of this technology—that is, those that are unconventional and unintended.

Proponents of nanotechnology predict that it will create many jobs. That means large numbers of people will be working with these materials. We must have a framework to address the occupational impacts of nanotechnology on human health.

Vicki Colvin
Director, Center for Biological and Environmental Nanotechnology
at Rice University
Professor of Chemistry, Rice University

A central question for toxicologists is how nanomaterials interact with biological materials. The chemical and physical composition and structure of engineered nanomaterials such as quantum dots are precisely defined. Most are highly pure and highly crystalline, with huge surface areas and a thick organic coating. These attributes, including size, play a critical role in the biological properties of these materials. However, testing their toxicity is challenging because such materials have various dimensions and properties, such as size, shape, and surface charge density.

This means that focusing on the toxicity of final nanoscale products will not work because there are too many parameters to control. Researchers must rethink their approach to evaluating the toxicity of these materials. This is especially critical because of their numerous medical applications, and the need to ensure public confidence in them.

For example, the features of engineered nano carbon 60—also known as fullerenes and carbon nanotubes—are very different from those of the aerosol nanoparticles used in many pulmonary studies of the toxicity of nanomaterials. Carbon 60 (C_{60}) can be used in a broad range of products, including anti-aging cream. However, one of the biggest applications may be in fuel cells, in which C_{60} allows for more efficient electron transfer. The question then becomes: Does the toxicity of C_{60} resemble that of molecular systems or soot, or is the toxicity entirely different? It turns out that putting carbon into a cage gives it unusual chemical properties that lead to distinctive biological impacts.

To evaluate such effects, Dr. Colvin's lab used in vitro experiments to examine the cytotoxicity of different forms of C_{60}. That is, what dose kills half the cells in a 48-hour exposure? The investigators found that although C_{60} is chemically inert, its chemical and physical properties make it highly biologically active, and very toxic in cell culture, although they wouldn't have predicted that result.

Why is that true? Small sizes lead to movement across cellular barriers, and toxicologists don't yet know the size cutoff above which such translocations do not occur. This produces high concentrations and strong interactions within cell membranes, generating free radicals and thus creating damage. Therefore, nanomaterials, designed to have very special chemical properties, can lead to adverse biological impacts.

Still, extrapolating to other nanomaterials is difficult. We could create thousands of dose-response curves for thousands of permutations of nanotubes. And toxicologists don't yet know what final nanoscale products will take the form of and what properties they possess. Thus, obtaining voluminous toxicological data is less useful than understanding the fundamental correlations between specific features of nanomaterials and their biological properties.

Surfaces are the vehicle for making these correlations. If chemists change the surface chemistry of C_{60}, they find that it can be virtually nontoxic. For example, the dose-response curves show that in a hydroxylated state, C_{60} is nontoxic up to the limits of solubility. However, when aggregated into dry powder, it is highly toxic. The material's biological impact—and its toxicity—depend on its surface and coating as well as its other features such as impurity levels.

If we understand why a material is cytotoxic, we should be able to make it less reactive and knock out its toxicity by systematically breaking its carbon bonds and oxidizing it. Thus, if fullerenes are used in fuel cells, they should be oxidized before they are dumped into the environment. This would eliminate their cytotoxicity and adverse effects on aquatic systems.

The debate isn't over whether nanomaterials are dangerous; some forms almost certainly are. At this early stage, we need to determine what strategies we can adopt to minimize these materials' toxicological activities. That means toxicology and nanotechnology should not proceed under business as usual, with toxicology used as the gate at the end of the process. Instead, chemists making systematic changes in materials must work with people who can measure their biological effects. Tight collaboration between materials engineers, chemists, and toxicologists could provide the essential data that can enable us to engineer safer nanomaterials from the beginning.

One of NNI's central challenges is to transform these multiple disciplines into a new one. To realize that goal, we need to recognize that the surfaces of nanomaterials have a more important impact than their composition in determining toxicity, and that toxicity can be turned on and off depending on surface coating. Forging any new discipline that combines two scientific languages is difficult. However, we must foster collaboration between particle toxicologists and nanotechnologists to provide the systematic information to ensure that the materials that drive the nanotechnology revolution are the safest we know how to make.

David Warheit
Toxicologist, DuPont Haskell Laboratory

The common perception is that nanoparticles (less than 100 nm) are always more toxic—in producing inflammation and fibrosis in the lungs of animals—than fine particles (100 nm to 3 microns) of similar composition. This notion is based on systematic studies of two types of particles: titanium dioxide and carbon black. (Diesel particles are also known to be toxic, but they have no nanoscale counterparts.)

Studies comparing the impact of nanoscale and fine particles on the lungs of rats can test this assumption. Researchers from Dr. Warheit's lab worked with toxicologists at Rice University to study the impact on rat lungs of exposure (by instillation) to fine-sized titanium oxide particles and nanoscale titanium oxide rods and dots. The study, which included two different doses, found that all the instilled particles caused an inflammatory response after 24 hours, indicating that all were initially inflammogenic. However, after this initial response subsided, the nanoparticles proved to be no more toxic than the fine-scaled particles after 1 week, 1 month, and 3 months post exposure. This occurred despite the fact that the nanodots had surface areas nearly 30 times larger than surface area of the fine-scaled titanium oxide.

In another study, the researchers compared the effects of fine-sized and nanoscale quartz particles, or crystalline silica, as that material is known to be particularly toxic. The study hypothesized that the nanoparticles would be even more toxic than fine-sized particles of identical composition at similar doses (although this dogma usually applies to low-solubility materials that are less toxic than the quartz). The researchers initially found that the nanoscale quartz particles were less toxic than the fine-scale particles. However, when they repeated the study, they found that the smallest nanoscale particles were more toxic than the fine-sized particles.

Workers tend to experience metal-fume fever for 24-48 hours after continuous high-level exposures to zinc oxide. The researchers therefore studied the effects of inhaled fine-scale and nanoscale zinc oxide on rat lungs. This study found no difference in the impact of the two different sizes of particles after 1 and 3 hours.

Many particles used in commerce are coated, so workers and consumers would be exposed to them in that form. Thus, another study by the same researchers examined the impact of titanium oxide particles when coated with various formulas of alumina and amorphous silica. This study found that different coatings can modify the length of time over which titanium oxide remains toxic in the lung. This finding underscores the importance of surface coatings in determining the health effects of particles.

The researchers concluded that the health impacts of nanoparticles must be evaluated on a case-by-case basis, as health risk is a product of hazard plus exposure. The health effects of nanoparticles will reflect their number, shape, and composition (whether they are crystalline or amorphous); their surface area, charge, and composition; the method by which they are synthesized (gas or liquid phase), and whether they aggregate. If the chemistry of particles differs, their biological effects may also differ. However, it is wrong to assume that nanoparticles are always more toxic than their fine-scale counterparts.

SESSION III:
ESTABLISHING STANDARDS AND GUIDELINES FOR
RESPONSIBLE ECONOMIC DEVELOPMENT

Jack Solomon
Praxair, retired

The NNI–Chemical Industry Consultative Board for Advancing Nanotechnology (CBAN) formed in March 2004 to promote collaborative industry-government R&D. CBAN has produced the "Nanomaterials by Design Roadmap" and established several working groups. One working group—composed of representatives from industry, academia, and federal agencies—focuses on the R&D needed to evaluate environmental, health, and safety (EHS) issues, especially by companies that want to commercialize nanotechnology.

Such research is critical because we lack methods and data on how best to develop nanomaterials and understand their EHS implications. We need a plan for assessing those impacts, and a funding structure that assigns clear responsibility for doing so to specific groups. Without such a plan, researchers may work on individual pieces of the EHS picture but fail to answer fundamental questions.

As an important first step, the CBAN working group and Oak Ridge National Laboratory have spearheaded creation of a database of existing information on the health, safety, and environmental effects of nanotechnology. Rice University has agreed to assume responsibility for maintaining this database, as it expands from an initial 1,200 articles to more than 8,000, and to ensure Web-based access. This database can become a clearinghouse for new information on nanomaterials and the routes of human and environmental exposure as it becomes available.

The EHS working group recommends further R&D in three core areas: the toxicity of nanomaterials; techniques for measuring and detecting them; and approaches to protecting the people who work with them and ensuring overall industrial hygiene. Specific needs include determining the best metrics for assessing the toxicity of nanoparticles, to ensure that the results are comparable; and developing a testing strategy, to ensure that we are investigating the materials that people will actually be exposed to.

Although we should use caution in generalizing about the toxicity of nano-materials, we cannot measure the EHS effects of thousands of individual particles. Thus we also need to select representative nanomaterials for testing. We further need a preliminary hazard assessment tool that can shed more light on exposure through inhalation, absorption via the skin, and oral ingestion, and compare the health and safety impacts to those of macroscale particles. For example, will the use of nanoscale iron to remediate contaminated groundwater risk exposing people through inhalation? Specific areas of research include determining the major factors that cause pulmonary toxicity, and weighing the health effects of inhaled particles on the brain.

We need to determine whether we can apply techniques for measuring bulk materials to nanomaterials, including whether electron beams, microscopy, and spectroscopy have nanoscale resolution. We also need to develop and verify tools for collecting and measuring samples of nanoparticles from soil, water, and air, to facilitate both short-term and long-term monitoring. We further must develop and validate methods for measuring biological activity linked with nanoparticles, including how they pass through cell membranes and dissolve in water and biological fluids. And we need to develop automated methods for screening and analyzing many different particles.

To ensure worker protection, we need to survey techniques for monitoring and analyzing workplace exposure to determine whether they are adequate for nanoparticles. Depending on the results, we may need to develop new air-sampling techniques, perhaps drawing on existing schemes now used in the semiconductor industry. We must also determine whether commercially available techniques for controlling air pollution during manufacturing—as well as standard protective equipment for workers—will get the job done. We further need to determine how nanoparticles released to the environment change over time, given changes in humidity, electrical fields, and temperatures.

Carol Henry
American Chemical Council

Although the potential benefits of nanotechnology are overwhelming, a key challenge is understanding its environmental, health, and safety (EHS) implica-tions. In pursuing that challenge we must examine the entire risk-benefit equation, because the unknowns concerning this technology are significant, and because history shows that public fears can inhibit a promising new technology. If we do not promote more interdisciplinary EHS research and better public communication of nanotechnology's risk and benefits, we will continue to repeat problems from the past. According to the U.S. Environmental Protection Agency, some 750 to 800 U.S.-based companies are already involved in nanotechnology. This number is likely to grow, along with increasing emphasis on better understanding of EHS implications.

Views of the EHS implications of nanotechnology range from "no problem" to "stop right here." However, closing off new nano-based approaches to remediating pollution because we are afraid of new risks would be a mistake. Instead, because of the arena's complexity, we must develop a rolling approach to characterizing risk that allows for interim decisions. We must also perform a gap analysis to determine the major EHS uncertainties, based on an inventory of existing research. The National Institute for Occupational Safety and Health has begun such an analysis.

Characterizing risk entails examining the entire exposure-dose-response cycle. This requires studying ecosystems as well as human health, identifying vulnerable populations, and investigating occupational, environmental, and consumer exposures. However, this task is formidable because we can make an infinite number of nanomaterials, and because we lack national and international risk-based standards and national and international research capacity for evaluating these materials. We must therefore develop more effective and efficient methods for studying exposure-dose-response pathways, and establish research priorities.

The highest near-term EHS priority is for methods for how to study these novel materials. At present, many public and private institutions are initiating research from their own perspective, with fundamental differences in approaches and without a framework for assessing or interpreting risks.

The United States needs a national strategy to avoid duplication of research and to set priorities. However, an international strategy would be even more effective, because nanomaterials, companies, and markets do not respect national boundaries. We also need an international clearinghouse to share and leverage knowledge and foster a cross-disciplinary focus. This will require more than just a website: the federal government must make active efforts to communicate information on potential risks and approaches to avoiding or mitigating them to developers, manufacturers, and the public, and to engage them in dialog. Annual workshops designed to facilitate the exchange of new knowledge on the EHS implications of nanotechnology could prove invaluable.

Major nanotechnology producers are actively trying to avoid risks to workers and consumers, such as by developing an occupational air-monitoring program. Industry does not shy away from regulations designed to protect the public and the environment, as that approach provides a more stable business climate. However, federal agencies must encourage academic laboratories and start-up companies to follow EHS approaches used by established manufacturers.

The National Nanotechnology Initiative is well situated to promote a collaborative approach and better communication between nanotechnologists and the EHS community. Toward that end efforts are needed under the NNI to publicly identify all existing and proposed EHS research, including at national laboratories, and to clarify whether such research is addressing implications or applications. Beyond that, while federal agencies have funded some research on the EHS implications of nanotechnology, they need to support far more, especially on fundamental methodological issues. If we let such critical research lag technological development, we will have learned little from past experience.

Lori Perine
American Forest and Paper Association

The U.S. forest products industry—which accounts for 7 percent of the U.S. manufacturing base and employs 1.3 million people—is a relative newcomer to nanotechnology. However, the industry is now aiming to use existing and emerging nanotechnology to improve today's products and processes, while also exploiting the nanoscale properties of cellulose fibrils to create new materials and products. In fact, nanotechnology promises to remake the industry by bolstering its financial performance while improving its energy efficiency and reducing its environmental impact.

The industry held its first workshop on how best to pursue these opportunities in October 2004, and it issued a roadmap in April 2005. The industry is now trying to build support for its research agenda and priorities among potential partners in government, academia, and other industries.

Cellulose has interesting properties at the sub-micro level, and its nanofibrils are extremely strong, holding 25 percent of the strength of carbon nanotubes. However, the industry does not yet know how to liberate these properties. Yet new analytical techniques are revealing the potential for lignocellulose—nature's nanobiomaterial and molecular-assembly machine—to become multifunctional and interact with other nanomaterials.

For example, if we can better understand and exploit the architecture and self-assembly of plant cell walls, we can grow cellulose nanomaterials with unique properties. These materials could provide breakthrough surface characteristics and bonding, serving as a matrix for other materials and allowing easy reconfiguration into other shapes and forms. Potential applications include novel biopolymers and other materials that are tailored to specific uses and are renewable, recyclable, and biodegradable.

Nanoscale cellulose materials could be used in composites with other materials to mitigate environmental, health, and safety concerns. This area shows promise because paper products are already used extensively in conjunction with medicine and food, and the properties of cellulose are generally compatible with human health and the environment.

The industry is already using existing nanotechnology to a limited extent. Printing speeds in modern pulp mills continue to rise, and consumers are demanding sharper colors; silica nanoparticles are enhancing performance in these areas by improving print quality. The industry is also using silicon nanoparticles to improve paper bags; nanosizing to improve products' surface properties; and nanoscale lime particles to stabilize 19th-century books.

Emerging nanotechnology offers the opportunity to monitor processes and products and revolutionize the pulp separations critical to manufacturing. For example, nanotechnology could enhance the dewatering process, help delignify wood, reduce the need for energy used in drying, and curb production of volatile organic compounds—major challenges in the industry. Nanosensors in intelligent wood and paper products could detect loads, moisture levels, and temperatures.

Nanotechnology further promises to enable the industry to make lighter-weight products from less material. Wood could also be engineered at the nanoscale to produce pharmaceutical products and to optimize the production of pulp, paper, and biofuel. Potential products include new wood preservatives and fire retardants.

To exploit these possibilities, we need to better understand the complexity and surface features of nanofibrils. The industry's priority areas for R&D include:

- Developing instrumentation and analytical techniques for characterizing cellulose nanostructures;
- Using existing nanomaterials, nanosensors, and other applications to improve the efficiency of converting raw materials into products, and to boost their performance;
- Using self-assembly of nanoscale building blocks in materials, structures, and coatings;
- Biofarming cellulose materials with unique multifunctional properties;
- Developing biomimetic processes for synthesizing cellulose-based nanomaterials;
- Manipulating tree genetics and cellular biology, chemistry, and physics to produce biological versions of carbon tubes;
- Developing multifunctional, self-assembling biopolymers that serve as unique nanomaterials and devices;
- Investigating the convergence of biopolymer nanostructures with silicon-based information technology in trees;
- Adapting nanomanufacturing technologies to cellulose surfaces;
- Exploring the use of nanocellulose materials in medical applications; and

- Exploring the efficient conversion of cellulose to renewable biofuels and biochemicals.

Through its Agenda 2020, the industry is beginning to form partnerships with federal and state governments, academia, and other industries to pursue this agenda. The industry is also considering whether it needs to adapt its existing environmental, health, and safety guidelines to address nanotechnology, perhaps learning from other materials-based industries.

Stephen Harper
Intel

More than 40 years ago, Gordon Moore, an Intel founder, accurately predicted the dramatic, sustained rise in the density of transistors on computer chips, accompanied by a radical reduction in their costs. Ambitious projects such as mapping the human genome and modeling proteins—as well as other cutting-edge applications of science and technology—depend on such rapid increases in affordable computational power.

Intel introduced nanofeatures—transistors less than 100 nanometers wide—into its products 5 years ago. A Pentium 4 chip now packs 100 million transistors, while the Itanium 2 chip includes 1.7 billion devices. Transistors 35 to 65 nanometers wide are now ready for mass-production. Because these nanoelectronics use traditional materials such as silicon, they are evolutionary, and their environmental, health, and safety issues are well understood.

To sustain Moore's law, research on new transistors is now focusing on the 10-nanometer scale (for comparison, DNA is 2 nanometers wide), with production expected in 2011. However, at that scale, the industry must rely on new nanomaterials such as carbon nanotubes and nanowires. These materials represent a greater leap, and their EHS risks are unknown. More research on these risks is therefore critical before the industry uses them in high-performance settings.

Two needs are common to all industries that will use nanotechnology: a better understanding of the toxicity of nanomaterials, and standard techniques for measuring and mitigating EHS concerns. Such research must be noncompetitive: that is, it must represent a collaborative effort among academia, government, nongovernmental organizations, and industry. This EHS research must develop common terminology and methods for assessing toxicity. It must also investigate exposure routes, pulmonary toxicology, other organ-specific toxicology, environmental toxicity, and the fate of nanomaterials. Specific EHS needs include methods for monitoring exposure, limits on exposure, engineering and protocols for personal protective equipment, and techniques for controlling emissions.

Intel collaborates with other companies such as DuPont in benchmarking EHS activities and also asks its university suppliers, as well as nanotech start-ups in which it is investing, to adhere to its EHS standards. However, the industry is unsure if today's techniques for addressing EHS concerns are adequate for nanotechnology

To support the needed research, Intel participates in the NNI and is a founding sponsor of the International Council on Nanotechnology, whose mission includes EHS concerns. Intel is also participating in nano-related activities of the American National Standards Institute and ASTM, and the Nanomaterial Handling Working Group of the National Institute for Occupational Safety and Health. The company aims to use the most conservative approach in protecting its employees—especially as any EHS-related disruptions in billion-dollar chip-fabricating plants can prove extremely costly. However, research must shed more light on what the best approach to protecting health and safety should be.

SESSION IV
DEFENSIVE TECHNOLOGIES, HUMAN ENHANCEMENT, AND ETHICAL ISSUES

George Khushf
Humanities Director, Center for Bioethics
Associate Professor of Philosophy, University of South Carolina

Bioethical debate traditionally distinguishes between medical interventions used for therapeutic reasons and those designed to enhance human form or function. Examples of the latter—where medicine reaches beyond its traditional domain—include sports doping, pharmaceuticals that bolster cognitive ability, and cosmetic surgery. Many developments associated with nanotechnology expand our capacity for enhancing human form and function, and they do this in ways that blur the line between therapy and enhancement. Nanotechnology, therefore, forces us to frame the ethical debate over how to proceed in a new way, and we are still struggling to find the appropriate terms for thinking through what is at stake.

The Nanotechnology, Biotechnology, Information Technology, and Cognitive Science Convergence project offers an example. This broad public-private initiative is designed to spur integration of four domains—nanotechnology, biotechnology, information technology, and cognitive science—within a 10 to 20-year time frame. Goals of the project include high-speed, broadband interface between brains and machines, and interventions that make the body more durable, energetic, easier to repair, and resistant to threats and the aging process. The initiative also aims to control the genetics of humans, animals, and agricultural plants, and it promises to tightly integrate the individual with the community. MIT's Institute for

Soldier Nanotechnologies contemplates a similarly radical enhancement of human capacity. The question is not just whether these outcomes might occur, but when and how. We already have teams of brilliant scientists funded to accomplish these goals. We now need to ask whether we have sufficiently reflected on the ethical issues integral to these projects.

These developments are more extreme than bioethics usually contemplates, with no clear line between conventional medical treatment and enhancement. The initiatives, therefore, argue for integrating ethical reflection into the R&D process—that is, to anticipate where we are going rather than simply reacting—to ensure that humanity benefits from such research.

At times, the diffuse and science-fiction-like character of these enhancements makes specifying and addressing ethical issues difficult. What's more, there is inherent tension between the desire to narrow NNI's participants' focus to define nanotechnology more carefully and the goal of expanding our thinking to address the profound ethical issues provoked by human enhancement. If we simply consider each piece of this picture separately, we won't see the radical extension of human capacities on the horizon.

The traditional model for addressing the social impacts of new technology assumes a neat divide between fundamental research and development on the one hand and ethics on the other, with the latter coming into play at the end of the process. Under this approach, ethics often involves a quasi-scientific process that relies on cost-benefit analysis, risk assessment, and risk communication, with broader concerns rationalized into a utility calculus. This model assumes a linear division of labor, in which we know who does what at each step. Facts and values are separate, risks and benefits are commensurable and scalable, and uncertainty can be understood and managed scientifically. In this model, proponents of a technology view public involvement as interference with the scientific process, and they focus on the adverse impacts of regulation.

However, when an emergent technology is radically disruptive, as some nanotechnology-based enhancements promise to be, we need to reconsider all facets of this model. Dr. Colvin provided a good example when she considered how an understanding of the relationship between the structure and the function of nanomaterials requires a new relationship between chemists and toxicologists. We need to extend such collaboration beyond two scientific disciplines to include people within the humanities as well as the sciences who desire to address the ethical and policy issues on the near-term horizon. We also need to develop guidelines for responsible conduct of researchers who go beyond therapeutics and want to enhance human abilities. We must also create an integrated approach to ethical issues, as a simple pro-versus-con debate will not help people think through the implications of nanotechnology-based human enhancement.

Rosalyn W. Berne
Associate Professor of Ethics and Religious Studies,
Department of Science, Technology, and Society, University of Virginia

Ethics seeks to identify principles that govern human choices and behaviors. Technological development, in contrast, focuses on solving perceived problems and improving the material conditions under which humans live. Military technology, in particular, is concerned with establishing power and control over forces deemed to be a threat.

Some 26 to 32 percent of NNI funds are devoted to achieving military ends. Specific projects include pulse-energy projectile weapons that seek to inflict severe pain from a distance, radar-resistant materials for use in unpiloted vehicles, sensors to detect biological and chemical toxins, technologies that extend the physical abilities of the soldier, and composite fabrics that can resist chemical and biological agents. These projects are based on the widely held notion that the nation is at risk from biological, chemical, radiological, and nuclear weapons. They also reflect the fact that as a nation, we feel vulnerable to destruction from any direction by myriad forces. The ultimate goal is to reduce casualties among our soldiers while ensuring swifter and more efficient destruction and death for others, that is, to become the most powerful force on the planet.

Nanoethics seek to understand the values and beliefs embedded in this quest for military dominance and to steer development of nanotechnology toward humanitarian aims. Yet these fundamental goals conflict with each other. Thus, the challenges of framing an ethics of military nanotechnology are formidable. How do we untangle these ideological conflicts and think through their ethical implications?

We could start by viewing military ethics through a three-dimensional framework. These three dimensions include practical concerns; questions about what constitutes morality in developing nanotechnology for military use; and metaethics, which seeks to elevate the psychological underpinnings of military nanotechnology from the tacit to the explicit.

The first dimension includes investigations into the potential toxicity of nanotechnology. We expect scientists and engineers to avoid exposing themselves and others to nanomaterials that might prove hazardous, and to avert irreversible environmental harm. However, we have only preliminary notions of which nanomaterials and devices could prove harmful, and information on health and safety hazards is so far inconclusive. Basic research, therefore, entails fundamental risks. The practical first dimension of military ethics also focuses on access—how to keep powerful new technologies out of the hands of others.

Second-dimension ethics asks what kinds of weapons and systems we ought to develop, and under what conditions we should use them. Such ethics would also ask: Who will provide the specialized retraining needed to operate these new systems? What kind of quality of life and economic opportunities will training and access provide, and for whom?

Second-dimension nanoethics would further ask: What is the best way for human beings to address disputes, and how can we distinguish right from wrong in the pursuit of military power? Sophisticated materials may ensure fewer casualties for our soldiers in the short term, but they may also may mean swifter death for others. Nanomaterials and devices are also likely to further erode rules for a fair battlefield, and may well prove a threat to ourselves in the long run.

Nanotechnology is often couched as an international contest; leaders have pointed to great economic opportunities if the United States wins the nanotech race. However, this notion, too, raises important second-dimension questions: Should the scientific process ever be rushed, and toward what end? What does it mean for people and nations to come in first? Technologies that offer the potential to restructure the body also provoke questions about how far we should alter human limits on physical power and longevity. And is controlling human existence with ever greater precision more important than solving other challenges, such as ensuring universal access to potable water? What will become of privacy and freedom in a nanotechnology-driven world? Will government use nanotechnology to assert a right to ubiquitous but invisible surveillance?

The Institute for Soldier Nanotechnology at MIT conceives the fact that soldiers carry too much weight and do not have enough protection as the central problems. Researchers hope to create strong, lightweight materials that protect soldiers better while improving their mobility. First-dimension nanoethics would see little dispute over the need to protect soldiers and support their work. However, the second dimension would pose ideological questions: Under which conditions is war just? Who decides questions concerning the taking and protecting of life?

The second dimension would also note that the resources society devotes to military applications of nanotechnology have ethical implications. For example, NNI is devoting not one dollar to eliminating war or devising technological solutions to the causes of war. Such concerns are always implicit in ethical considerations of war. However, each advance in efficiency and sophistication strengthens humanity's capacity for more profound destruction, and thus nanotechnology forces us to actively address such implications.

A key third-dimension question concerns the connection between human psychological makeup and the pursuit of military power and dominance through nanotechnology. This approach would consider claims of disease control, beliefs about material existence, and the fear of death. The third dimension would also consider the role of metaphor in creating meaning.

In fact, the imaginative dimensions of morality are critical. For example, how might moral imagination prompt us to turn the military uses of nanotechnology toward preserving human life and the planet? If ethics can expand our moral imagination, might we conceive—instead of a nanojet fighter—a nanojet immobilizer that renders bombs and missiles totally powerless?

SESSION V
SOCIETAL IMPLICATIONS OF NANOTECHNOLOGY

Jane Macoubrie
Embry Research and Communications, Denver, Colorado
Senior Advisor to Project on Emerging Nanotechnologies,
Woodrow Wilson International Center for Scholars

From 2001 forward, an interdisciplinary team of social scientists at North Carolina State University has conducted several "citizen consensus conferences"—based on a Danish model—and other studies aimed at testing and creating mechanisms for effective public participation in U.S. technology policymaking. Citizen consensus conferences always include citizen recommendations to government. The first such conference in 2001 was held in face-to-face mode, on the topic of genetically modified foods. A second conference was held wholly via group conferencing software on the Internet. And in 2003, we held several more conferences to further test the Internet-mediated approach, this time focusing on the topic of global warming.

In 2004, two of us conducted the first demographically representative national survey of public awareness of and attitudes toward nanotechnology. Additionally, I developed and separately convened experimental issue groups (EIGs), in which participants received information on different development scenarios for nanotechnology and then reported their views on benefits and expressed their concerns.

Of the 1,536 people who participated in the national survey, we found that 52 percent had heard "nothing" about nanotechnology, while 32 percent had heard "a little." We also found that only 16 percent had heard "quite a bit" or "a lot." Just 3 percent could answer three true-or-false questions about the technology correctly, while 34 percent could answer two questions correctly. However, 40 percent thought the benefits of nanotechnology would outweigh the risks, while 38 percent thought risks and benefits would be about equal.

From data gathered via the experimental issue groups, I found that participants ranked "reduced health casualties" as the primary gain they hoped for from nanotechnology—which included finding better cures for major diseases, developing less invasive treatments with fewer side effects, and taking care of basic health care needs such as cavities. Participants cited environmental cleanup and protection as the next most important desired benefit from nanotechnology, followed by better jobs and a stronger economy, better consumer products, and new materials for exploring deep space and water. They also hoped for higher-quality food, options for repairing and regenerating the body, and solutions to world problems such as desalinization, food, transportation, and energy.

Participants in the groups cited military uses—including the potential for another arms race, more terrorism, and more pollution of military bases—as the most important anticipated downsides of nanotechnology. They also expressed concern about its long-term health effects and environmental footprint. However, the broadest area of concern involved nanotechnology's social footprint, which included a potential loss of freedom of choice and privacy, a loss of control by regulators, and ethical challenges.

At least two-thirds of both survey respondents and group participants do not trust government or industry leaders to manage these risks effectively. Participants with a college degree or higher expressed the lowest level of trust. Participants were most concerned about the ability of government to manage the risks of nano-technology in medicine and industrial arenas—with the former an unexpected concern.

The EIG study also investigated the reasoning underlying people's attitudes toward nanotechnology. I found that participants based their concerns largely on experience rather than fears of out-of-control nano-robots. Indeed, they already see a lack of control and tracking of the risks of nanotechnology. The bottom line is that the public is excited about the promise of nanotechnology but wants to know how it will be managed.

These results suggest that mechanisms soliciting citizens' views on the most desired benefits and unwanted risks of technology can provide important infor-mation not available elsewhere. However, to obtain valid and replicable results for citizen forums, organizers must develop a consistent process for convening them, including a uniform process for recruiting participants and creating briefing mate-rials, and metrics for measuring effectiveness. Some known processes create greater polarization of views, for examples and others lead to great citizen frustration. Neither is a desirable outcome, as both worsen citizen perceptions of and levels of trust in government.

Although conducting citizen technology forums is challenging, ensuring a public voice in technology policy is critical. We need both evolutionary and revo-lutionary mechanisms for soliciting greater public input—beyond established interest groups—and for giving citizens a seat at the policymaking table.

Note: Since this workshop, Dr. Macoubrie was lead author of a paper entitled "Informed Public Perceptions of Nanotechnology and Trust in Government" released in 2005 by the Project on Emerging Nanotechnologies from the Woodrow Wilson International Center for Scholars and the Pew Charitable Trusts. The report is based on a study conducted to assess general public perceptions, which provided evidence of support for nanotechnology and its benefits, more public involvement in information sharing about nanotechnology products and developments, and a general mistrust of the government to manage technology-related risks. She also has published "Nanotechnology: Public Concerns, Reasoning, and Trust in Government" (J. Macoubrie. 2006. Nanotechnology: Public concerns, reasoning, and trust in government. Public Understanding of Science 15:221-241), a report on a 2004 experimental issue group study of concerns about and expectations for nanotechnology.

Kristen Kulinowski
Faculty Fellow of Chemistry, Rice University
Executive Director for Policy
Center for Biological and Environmental Nanotechnology, Rice University

As nanomaterials begin to appear in consumer products amid talk about the potential for controlling disease, protecting soldiers, and facilitating exploration of deep space, civil society groups are focusing on the environmental, health, and safety implications of these uses. Many scientists are concerned that experience with nanotechnology will parallel that with genetically modified foods and other technologies, with early enthusiasm vanishing as health and environmental concerns emerge, prompting a backlash against widespread use. Indeed, some of the same players that oppose nuclear power and agricultural biotechnology are beginning to address the risks of nanotechnology. For example, Greenpeace has called for a moratorium on further nanotechnology research until the hazards are better understood and laboratory controls are in place.

The combination of many concerned stakeholders and numerous unanswered social and environmental questions has strong potential to result in confusion and misinformation. Social science researchers are performing well-documented studies of public perceptions of nanotechnology. However, to avoid the familiar "wow-to-yuck" trajectory, the Center for Biological and Environmental Nanotechnology (CBEN) sees a need to engage the public in policy interactions with government and industry, and to incorporate nanotechnology into the curriculum at all educational levels. These efforts should include inviting public interest groups and citizens to participate in roadmapping workshops for nanotechnology.

Toward that end, CBEN has created the International Council on Nanotechnology (ICON) to "assess, communicate, and reduce the environmental and health risks of nanotechnology." ICON includes representatives from academia, government, nongovernmental groups, and companies from numerous industrial sectors. ICON is based on a network model, to enable all these stakeholders to interact. The idea emanated partly from conversations with CBEN's industrial affiliates, who worry that environmental, health, and safety concerns will add risk to their investments in nanotechnology.

ICON is focusing on research on both the technical and the social risks of nanotechnology, developing standards, and creating unbiased information for the lay public. As one piece of these efforts, ICON is working with CBEN to post a comprehensive database of nanotechnology-related research on the Web, and to include lay summaries of important findings and place them in their larger context.

However, such efforts need to move beyond simply assessing risk in the laboratory to consider more fundamental social and political questions. These include: Why this technology? Who needs it? Who benefits from it? Who is controlling it? Can developers be trusted? What will it mean for me and my family? Will it improve the environment? And how will it affect people in the developing world? All these questions must be part of the risk-assessment landscape.

To encourage college students to address these questions, CBEN developed an undergraduate course—funded by the National Science Foundation—to enable them to distinguish fact from fiction regarding nanotechnology, and to consider what role they will play in determining its future. As part of the course, each student testified before a mock city council—which was trying to decide whether to approve a nanotechnology laboratory—representing the position of a corporate leader, a nanotechnology expert, a environmental advocate, a government regulator, a worker, or a local community group. Teachers at other universities are developing similar courses designed to encourage students to actively weigh the future of nanotechnology.

Richard Denison
Senior Scientist, Environmental Defense

In the mid-1990s, Environmental Defense followed up on reports from the National Research Council (NRC) on the lack of information on high-volume industrial chemicals by working with the U.S. Environmental Protection Agency (EPA) and industry to generate better information and make it public. That effort provides a model for the constructive engagement needed to address the new class of chemical substances known as engineered nanomaterials.

Familiar materials can exhibit wholly new properties when reengineered at the nanoscale. For example, the same metallic aluminum used in soda cans can be used at the nanoscale as a catalyst in rocket fuel. Subtle differences in otherwise identical nanomaterials—such as the degree of twist in carbon nanotubes—can affect their electrical conductivity. The upside of these properties is an enormous range of possible applications, many with potential environmental and health benefits. However, the downside is the potential for some of those same materials to enter the environment and interact with living systems in ways that pose potential risks, including a range of toxicities. For example, preliminary studies suggest that some nanomaterials may cross the blood–brain barrier or accumulate in living tissue. If the public is not convinced that developers of this potentially transformative technology and their government overseers can manage these risks, we will see a significant backlash against them, paralleling that seen with genetically modified foods.

Most studies of the potential risks of nanotechnology have examined the impact of fairly high doses over short-term exposures. Because the results are preliminary, the need for more research is clear. However, until recently the government devoted just $10 million or less of the $1 billion spent annually on nanotechnology to risk-related studies. Federal agencies have since boosted their support for research on environmental, health, and safety risks to about $40 million. However, the federal government needs to devote at least $100 million annually for at least several years to better understand the implications side of the equation—a modest investment considering the magnitude of the challenge.[2]

The federal government must also perform other vital roles, including enhancing regulatory policies. The existing regulatory structure appears to have a number of gaps and loopholes. For example, because of the breadth of applications of nanotechnology, numerous federal agencies have potential jurisdiction, including the Occupational Safety and Health Administration, the Environmental Protection Agency, the Food and Drug Administration, and the Consumer Product Safety Commission. However, existing legislation allows some of these agencies to impose few requirements for pre-market testing, and so they can respond to problems mostly only after the fact. For example, the applicability of the Toxic Substances Control Act to nanomaterials is uncertain. If nanomaterials are considered new chemicals, then manufacturers must notify the EPA so it can evaluate the magnitude of the risks. However, if nanomaterials are considered existing materials, industry does not have to provide such notification. EPA has so far received only a small number of notifications from manufacturers. Confusion over nomenclature only complicates the task. These loopholes need to be closed and regulatory authority enhanced to allow adequate scrutiny of nanomaterials before they appear on

---

[2]See Environmental Defense's companion analysis, prepared at the request of and submitted to the NRC's Committee to Review the NNI, which provides a rationale for this proposal.

the market, as well as more interagency coordination and authority to address crosscutting impacts.

The first step is to acknowledge that nanomaterials differ from bulk materials. Industry and government authorities also need to adopt a life cycle approach to managing nanomaterials, take interim steps to manage risks before they are completely understood, and embrace public disclosure of all risk-related information. Responsible steps include assuming that such materials and wastes containing them are toxic until proven otherwise, monitoring workplaces, and requiring worker training and effective industrial hygiene.

The NNI's Nanoscale Science, Engineering and Technology (NSET) Subcommittee has a critical role to play in overseeing federal research dollars spent on health and environmental risks, and in performing a "gap analysis" of loopholes in federal oversight. To fulfill those roles, NSET should request and make public detailed information on federal agency plans for risk-related research and draw on the expertise of groups such as the NRC Board on Environmental Studies and Toxicology to help shape an overall strategy. NSET must also move beyond the traditional top-down approach, giving stakeholders such as workers, consumers, and health and environmental advocates a seat at the agenda-setting and policy-making table.

Dietram A. Scheufele
Professor, School of Journalism and Mass Communication and Department of Life Sciences Communication, University of Wisconsin, Madison

What does the public think, know, and feel about nanotechnology, and how does it form these attitudes? When we first proposed a longitudinal research project to NSF to investigate these questions, some reviewers raised the question whether assessing public opinion toward nanotechnology is even possible at this early stage. And the answer is simple: It is possible and necessary to understand how people form opinions about nanotech, *especially* in the absence of information. This thinking is based on two models for how laypeople obtain information and develop attitudes toward science and technology.

The first model focuses on scientific literacy. This model assumes that the public has relatively limited information on scientific issues but that attitudes toward science and scientists would be more favorable if people knew more about them. However, this model is based on one inherent fallacy: that if the public learned about evidence-based inquiry and peer-reviewed findings, it would come to the same conclusions as scientists. But this assumption, of course, is flawed for two reasons. First, most research does not show a consistent link between scientific literacy and support for emerging technologies—either positive or negative.

Second, if people made decisions based exclusively on facts, we would not need systematic rules of scientific inquiry in the first place.

The second model is called the "cognitive miser" model. It also holds that people know very little about most issues, but that it makes little sense for most people to develop in-depth understanding given the thousands of decisions they must make every day. However, people still form attitudes and opinions, often without having a comprehensive understanding of the issues. To do so, they rely on shortcuts and cues based on religion, ideology, coverage in the mass media, and the opinions of others, tapping these sources more heavily the less information they have. For example, entertainment media provide many people's understanding of how scientists work by cultivating certain images of scientists in movies and TV shows.

To investigate these models and better understand how people are beginning to form judgments about nanotechnology, we conducted a national survey of 706 respondents in 2004. We found that participants were most knowledgeable about the economic implications of nanotechnology, including the notion that it represents the next scientific revolution. We also found relatively high levels of basic knowledge, such as that nanomaterials are invisible to the human eye, and that nanotechnology allows modifications that do not occur in nature. However, people were less well informed about specific aspects of nanotechnology, such as the definition of a nanometer and its size compared with that of an atom.

People being interviewed who said they were aware of nanotechnology before were much more inclined to express overall support for its use than people who said they had been unaware of this new technology. However, we found no significant differences between aware and unaware respondents in their perception of the *risks* of nanotechnology. People in both groups expressed their deepest concern about potential loss of privacy, and also cited concern about a new arms race and a loss of U.S. jobs, expressing lowest concern about self-replicating robots. Still, we did find a significant difference between aware and unaware respondents regarding perceived *benefits*: the former were much more optimistic about the possibilities for cleaning up the environment, treating disease, improving national security, and enhancing human abilities.

The most obvious explanation is that people who were more optimistic about nanotechnology knew more about it. However, we did not find this interpretation to be supported by the data. Instead, we found that they relied more heavily on scientific media. These findings support the cognitve miser model. Specifically, what is the role of the media in influencing attitudes toward nanotechnology? Heavy users of science media may be more supportive of nanotechnology because coverage currently focuses mostly on its potential benefits rather than its risks. Today, a science writer does a majority of the reporting on nanotechnology for the

Washington Post, while the *New York Times* has assigned a business reporter to such coverage. Science and business media not only inform their audiences but likely "frame" nanotechnology positively.

Attitudes toward nanotechnology will change as mainstream media, rather than more specialized science and technology reporters, reframe the debate. Mainstream media will focus attention on potential downsides, and people will base their attitudes on the views of critics who cite the potential for toxic contamination and loss of privacy. Although public awareness and knowledge of nanotechnology will grow, attitudes will rest on packaging rather than content, as interest groups and policymakers offer competing frames. Scientifically based public discussion is unlikely to occur.

Further research on how people make decisions regarding nanotechnology is needed to answer several questions. What frames regarding nanotechnology now exist in the public arena, and what frames are likely to appear? How do these frames become part of the media agenda? What role can scientists, industry, and science writers play in influencing these dynamics? How will public opinion develop over the long term? Answering these questions is important because we do not fully understand how the public develops its attitudes and makes decisions regarding significant developments in science and technology as these issues emerge on the public agenda.

RELATED READING

Altmann, J., and M. Gubrud. 2004. Anticipating military nanotechnology. IEEE Technology and Society Magazine 21(4).

Balbus, J., R. Denison, K. Florini, and S. Walsh. 2005. Getting nanotechnology right the first time. Issues in Science and Technology (Summer):65-71.

Bergeron, S., and E. Archambault. 2005. Canadian Stewardship Practices for Environmental Nanotechnology.

Bergeson, L.L. 2006. Nanoscale materials and TSCA: EPA's NPPTAC recommends a framework for a voluntary program. Environmental Quality Management. Spring.

Bhattacharyya, D., W. Chen, G. Chumanov, V. Colvin, M.S. Diallo, J. Doshi, R.E. Gawley, M.V. Johnston, S.C. Larsen, T. Masciangioli, P.H. McMurray, A. Myers, P. Pascual, D. Rejelski, M. Roco, D. Rolison, S.I. Shah, W.Y. Shih, W.M. Sigmund, D.R. Strongin, T. Sun, N. Tao, W.C. Trogler, D. Velegol, M. Wiesner, X.D. Xiang, and W.X. Zhang. 2003. Nanotechnology and the Environment: Applications and Implications. STAR Progress Review Workshop, National Center for Environmental Research, Office of Research and Development, Environmental Protection Agency. Washington, D.C.: U.S. Environmental Protection Agency.

Cable, J. 2005. A best practices approach to minimizing EHS risk in nanotechnology manufacturing. Occupational Hazards. October 6. Available at http://www.occupationalhazards.com/articles/14129, accessed February 2006.

Colvin, V.L. 2003. The potential environmental impact of engineered nanomaterials. Nat. Biotechnol. 21(10): 1166-1170.

Crichton, M. 2002. Prey. HarperCollins.

Denison, Richard A., Environmental Defense. 2005. A proposal to increase federal funding of nanotechnology risk research to at least $100 million annually. Available at http://www.environmentaldefense.org/documents/4442_100milquestionl.pdf.

Doraiswamy, Krishna, Environmental and safety impacts of nanotechnology: What research is needed?, presentation made at U.S. House of Representatives Committee on Science Hearing, November 17, 2005. Available at http://commdocs.house.gov/committees/science/hsy24464.000/hsy24464_0.HTM.

Economic & Social Research Council. 2003. The Social and Economic Challenges of Nanotechnology. United Kingdom.

Elder, A., R. Gelein, M. Azadniv, M. Frampton, J. Finkelstein, and G. Oberdörster. 2004. Systemic effects of inhaled ultrafine particles in two compromised, aged rat strains. Inhalation Toxicology 16:461-471.

ETC Group. 2003. The Big Down: From Genomes to Atoms. Winnipeg, Manitoba: ETC Group.

ETC Group. 2004. Down on the Farm: The Impact of Nano-Scale Technologies on Food and Agriculture. Ottawa, Ontario: ETC Group. November.

European Commission (EC). 2003. The New EU Chemicals Legislation-REACH. Available at http://europa.eu.int/comm/enterprise/reach/index_en.htm.

European Commission (EC). 2004. Towards a European strategy for nanotechnology. Communication from the Commission of European Communities.

European Commission (EC). 2005. Nanoscience and nanotechnologies: An action plan for Europe 2005-2009. Communication from the Commission to the Council, the European Parliament and the Economic and Social Committee. July 6.

Fonash, S.J. 2001. Education and training of the nanotechnology workforce. J. Nanoparticle Res. 3:79-82.

Francesconi, R. 2004. Survey Shows Public Can Discern Nano's Benefits. Ann Arbor, Mich.: Small Times Media.

Friedman, S.M., and B.P. Egolf. 2005. Nanotechnology: Risks and the media. IEEE Technology and Society 24(Winter):5-11.

Greenpeace Environmental Trust. 2003. Future Technologies, Today's Choices. United Kingdom.

Hampton, T. 2005. Researchers size up nanotechnology risks. JAMA 294:1881-1883.

Hardman, R. 2006. A toxicologic review of quantum dots: Toxicity depends on physicochemical and environmental factors. Environmental Health Perspectives 114:165-172.

Health and Safety Executive. 2004. Health Effects of Particles Produced for Nanotechnologies. United Kingdom.

HM Government. 2005. Response to the Royal Society and the Royal Academy of Engineering Report: "Nanoscience and Nanotechnologies: Opportunities and Uncertainties." London: HM Government.

HM Government. 2005. Characterising the Potential Risks Posed by Engineered Nanoparticles. London: HM Government.

Hood, E. 2004. Nanotechnology: Looking as we leap. Environmental Health Perspectives 112:A740-A749.

Institute of Medicine. 2005. Implications of Nanotechnology for Environmental Health Research. Lynn Goldman and Christine Coussens, eds. Washington, D.C.: The National Academies Press.

Institute of Medicine and National Research Council. 2004. Safety of Genetically Engineered Foods: Approaches to Assessing Unintended Health Effects. Washington, D.C.: The National Academies Press.

International Risk Governance Council. 2006. Survey on Nanotechnology Governance. Volume A. The Role of Government. Geneva. January.

Joy, B. 2000. Why the future doesn't need us. Wired 8(04).

Kalpin, M.C., and M. Hoffer. 2005. Nanotechnology and the environment: Will emerging environmental regulations stifle the promise? NSTI Nanotech 2005 Conference and Trade Show, Anaheim, Calif., May 8-12, 2005.

Kurzweil, R. 1999. The Age of Spiritual Machines: When Computers Exceed Human Intelligence. Viking Adult.

Lam, C.-W., J.T. James, R. McCluskey, and R.L. Hunter. 2004. Pulmonary toxicity of single-wall carbon nanotubes in mice 7 and 90 days after intratracheal instillation. Toxicological Sciences 77:126-134.

Lewenstein, B.V. 2005. What counts as a "social and ethical issue" in nanotechnology? HYLE-International Journal for Philosophy of Chemistry 11:5-18.

Macoubrie, J. 2005. Informed Public Perceptions of Nanotechnology and Trust in Government. Washington, D.C.: Woodrow Wilson International Center for Scholars Project on Emerging Nanotechnologies.

Meridian Institute. 2004. Report of the International Dialogue on Responsible Research and Development of Nanotechnology.

Meridian Institute. 2005. Global Dialogue on Nanotechnology and the Poor: Opportunities and Risks. Available at http://www.nanoandthepoor.org.gdnp.php.

Nanoforum. 2005. Fourth Nanoforum Report: Benefits, Risks, Ethical, Legal and Social Aspects of Nanotechnology. Second Edition. For more information, see http://www.nanoforum.org.

Nanoscale Science, Engineering and Technology Subcommittee, Committee on Technology, National Science and Technology Council (NSTC). 2001. Societal Implications of Nanoscience and Nanotechnology. Washington, D.C.: NSTC.

Nanoscale Science, Engineering and Technology Subcommittee, Committee on Technology, National Science and Technology Council. 2005. The National Nanotechnology Initiative: Research and Development Leading to a Revolution in Technology and Industry. Supplement to the President's FY 2006 Budget Request. March.

Nanoscale Science, Engineering and Technology Subcommittee, Committee on Technology, National Science and Technology Council (NSTC). 2005. Regional, State, and Local Initiatives in Nanotechnology. Washington, D.C.: NSTC.

Nanoscale Science, Engineering and Technology Subcommittee, Committee on Technology, National Science and Technology Council (NSTC). 2005. Nanotechnology: Societal Implications—Maximizing Benefits for Humanity. Washington, D.C.: NSTC.

National Academy of Sciences, National Academy of Engineering, and Institute of Medicine. 2005. Rising Above the Gathering Storm: Energizing and Employing America for a Brighter Economic Future. (prepublication copy). Washington, D.C.: The National Academies Press.

National Institute for Occupational Safety and Health (NIOSH). 2005. Strategic Plan for NIOSH Nanotechnology Research: Filling the Knowledge Gaps. Washington, D.C.: NIOSH.

Nel, A.,T. Xia, L. Mädler, and N. Li. 2006. Toxic potential of materials at the nanolevel. Science 311:622-627.

Oberdörster, G., A. Maynard, K. Donaldson, V. Castranova, J. Fitzpatrick, K. Ausman, J. Carter, B. Karn,W. Kreyling, D. Lai, S. Olin, N. Monteiro-Riviere, D. Warheit, and H. Yang. 2005. Principles for characterizing the potential human health effects from exposure to nanomaterials: Elements of a screening strategy. Particle and Fibre Toxicology 2:8.

Phibbs, P. 2004. Nonprofit institute to work with industry, organizations to develop voluntary standards. Bureau of National Affairs, June 17, p. A-6.

Phoenix, C., and E. Drexler. 2004. Safe exponential manufacturing. Nanotechnology 15:869-872.

President's Council of Advisors on Science and Technology (PCAST). 2005. The National Nanotechnology Initiative at Five Years: Assessment and Recommendations of the National Nanotechnology Advisory Panel. Washington, D.C.: PCAST.

Rejeski, D. 2004. The next small thing. The Environmental Forum. Washington, D.C.: The Environmental Law Institute.

Reynolds, G.H. 2002. Forward to the Future: Nanotechnology and Regulatory Policy. San Francisco: Pacific Research Institute.

Reynolds, G.H. 2003. Nanotechnology and regulatory policy: Three futures. Harv. J. Law Technol. 17(1):180-209.

Royal Society and the Royal Academy of Engineering. 2004. Nanoscience and Nanotechnologies: Opportunities and Uncertainties. United Kingdom: Royal Society.

Royal Society and the Science Council of Japan. 2005. Report of a Joint Royal Society–Science Council of Japan Workshop on the Potential Health, Environmental and Societal Impacts of Nanotechnologies. United Kingdom: Royal Society.

Salamanca-Buentello, F., D.L. Persad, E.B. Court, D.K. Martin, A.S. Daar, and P.A. Singer. 2005. Nanotechnology and the developing world. PLoS Medicine 2(5):e97.

Semmler, M., J. Seitz, F. Erbe, P. Mayer, J. Heyder, G. Oberdörster, and W. Kreyling. 2004. Long-term clearance kinetics of inhaled ultrafine insoluble iridium particles from the rat lung, including transient translocation into secondary organs. Inhalation Toxicology 16:453-459.

Singer, P.A., F. Salamanca-Buentello, and A.S. Daar. 2005. Harnessing nanotechnology to improve global equity. Issues in Science and Technology (Summer):57-64.

Sternstein, A. 2005. EPA data littered with errors and gaps. August 24. Available at http://www.fcw.com/article90389-08-24-05-Web.

Swiss Re. 2004. Nanotechnology: Small Matter, Many Unknowns. Zurich, Switzerland: Swiss Reinsurance Company.

Toxic Substances Control Act (TSCA), 15 U.S.C. s/s 2601 et seq. 1976. Available at http://www.epa.gov/region5/defs/html/tsca.htm, accessed February 2006.

Toxic Substances Control Act (TSCA), 15 U.S.C. s/s 2602 (2)(a). 1976. Available at http://www.epa.gov/region5/defs/html/tsca.htm, accessed February 2006.

Toxic Substances Control Act (TSCA), 15 U.S.C. s/s 2602 (9). 1976. Available at http://www.epa.gov/region5/defs/html/tsca.htm, accessed February 2006.

U.S. Environmental Protection Agency. 2005. Nanotechnology white paper (external review draft). Available at http://www.epa.gov/osa/pdfs/EPA_nanotechnology_white_paper_external_review_draft_12-02-2005.pdf.

U.S. House of Representatives Committee on Science Hearing, The Societal Implications of Nanotechnology, April 9, 2003. Available at http://commdocs.house.gov/committees/science/hsy86340.000/hsy86340_0.HTM.

Warheit, D.B., B.R. Laurence, K.L. Reed, D.H. Roach, G.A.M. Reynolds, and T.R. Webb. 2004. Comparative pulmonary toxicity assessment of single-wall carbon nanotubes in rats. Toxicological Sciences 77:117-125.

Warner, J.C., A.S. Cannon, and K.M. Dye. 2004. Green chemistry. Environmental Impact Assessment Review 24:775-799.

Weiss, R. 2004. "Data Quality" law is nemesis of regulation. Washington Post, August 16.

Weiss, R. 2005. Nanotechnology regulation needed, critics say. Washington Post, December 5.

Wilsdon, J., and R. Willis. 2004. See-Through Science: Why Public Engagement Needs to Move Upstream. United Kingdom: Demos.

E

Acronyms

AAAS	American Association for the Advancement of Science
ANSI	American National Standards Institute
ASTM	American Society for Testing and Materials
BIS	Bureau of Industry and Security (Department of Commerce)
CBAN	Consultative Board for Advancing Nanotechnology
CBEN	Center for Biological and Environmental Nanotechnology
CDC	Centers for Disease Control and Prevention
CPSC	Consumer Product Safety Commission
CSREES	Cooperative State Research, Education, and Extension Service (USDA)
DHS	Department of Homeland Security
DNA	deoxyribonucleic acid
DOC	Department of Commerce
DOD	Department of Defense
DOE	Department of Energy
DOJ	Department of Justice
DOL	Department of Labor
DOT	Department of Transportation
DOTreas	Department of the Treasury

EC   European Commission
ED   Department of Education
EHS   environmental, health, and safety
EIG   experimental issue group
EPA   Environmental Protection Agency
EU   European Union

FDA   Food and Drug Administration
FHSA   Federal Hazardous Substances Act
FS   Forest Service

GNN   Global Nanotechnology Network (workshop)

HHS   Health and Human Services, Department of

IEEE   Institute of Electrical and Electronics Engineers
ISO   International Organization for Standardization
ITC   International Trade Commission
ITIC   Intelligence Technology Innovation Center
IWGN   Interagency Working Group on Nanotechnology

LCA   life cycle analysis

MOU   memorandum of understanding

NASA   National Aeronautics and Space Administration
NCI   National Cancer Institute
NCN   Network for Computational Nanotechnology
NEHI   Nanotechnology Environmental and Health Implications (working
            group of the NSET Subcommittee)
NGO   nongovernmental organization
NIEHS   National Institute of Environmental Health Sciences
NIH   National Institutes of Health
NIOSH   National Institute for Occupational Safety and Health
NIRT   Nanoscale Interdisciplinary Research Team (NSF program)
NIST   National Institute of Standards and Technology
NNAP   National Nanotechnology Advisory Panel
NNCO   National Nanotechnology Coordination Office
NNI   National Nanotechnology Initiative
NNIN   National Nanotechnology Infrastructure Network (NSF program)

NRC   National Research Council
NRL   Naval Research Laboratory
NSECs   Nanoscale Science and Engineering Centers (NSF program)
NSET   Nanoscale Science, Engineering, and Technology (Subcommittee of
            the NSTC)
NSF   National Science Foundation
NSP   Nanotechnology Standards Panel (ANSI)
NSRC   Nanoscale Science Research Centers (DOE program)
NSTC   National Science and Technology Council
NTP   National Toxicology Program
NTRC   Nanotechnology Research Center (NIOSH)

OMB   Office of Management and Budget
ORD   Office of Research and Development (EPA)
OSTP   Office of Science and Technology Policy

PCA   program component area
PCAST   President's Council of Advisors on Science and Technology

R&D   research and development
REACH   Registration, Evaluation and Authorisation of Chemicals

SBIR   Small Business Innovation Research (multiagency program)
STAR   Science to Achieve Results (program)
STEM   science, technology, engineering, and mathematics
STTR   Small Business Technology Transfer (multiagency program)
SWNT   single-wall carbon nanotube

TA   Technology Administration (Department of Commerce)
TAG   technical advisory group
TF   task force
TSCA   Toxic Substances Control Act

USDA   U.S. Department of Agriculture
U.S. NRC   U.S. Nuclear Regulatory Commission
USPTO   U.S. Patent and Trademark Office (Department of Commerce)

VC   venture capital

WG   working group